THE BEHAVIORAL AND SOCIAL SCIENCES SURVEY
Psychiatry Panel

David A. Hamburg, *Chairman*
Stanford University School of Medicine

Douglas Bond
Case Western Reserve University School of Medicine

Leon Eisenberg
Harvard Medical School and *Massachusetts General Hospital*

Roy R. Grinker, Sr.
*Michael Reese Hospital and Medical Center and
Pritzler School of Medicine, University of Chicago*

F. C. Redlich
Yale University School of Medicine

Melvin Sabshin
University of Illinois College of Medicine

Albert Stunkard
University of Pennsylvania School of Medicine

SC 71

PSYCHIATRY AS A BEHAVIORAL SCIENCE

Edited by
David A. Hamburg

A SPECTRUM BOOK

Prentice-Hall, Inc., *Englewood Cliffs, N. J.*

Current printing (last number):
10 9 8 7 6 5 4 3 2 1

Prentice-Hall International, Inc. (*London*)
Prentice-Hall of Australia, Pty. Ltd. (*Sydney*)
Prentice-Hall of Canada, Ltd. (*Toronto*)
Prentice-Hall of India Private Limited (*New Delhi*)
Prentice-Hall of Japan, Inc. (*Tokyo*)

FOREWORD

This book is one of a series prepared in connection with the Survey of the Behavioral and Social Sciences conducted between 1967 and 1969 under the auspices of the Committee on Science and Public Policy of the National Academy of Sciences and the Problems and Policy Committee of the Social Science Research Council.

The Survey provides a comprehensive review and appraisal of these rapidly expanding fields of knowledge, and constitutes a basis for an informed, effective national policy to strengthen and develop these fields even further.

The reports in the Survey, each the work of a panel of scholars, include studies of anthropology, economics, geography, history as a social science, political science, psychology, psychiatry as a behavioral science, sociology, and the social science aspects of statistics, mathematics and computation. A general volume, *The Behavioral and Social Sciences: Outlook and Needs* (Englewood Cliffs, N. J.: Prentice-Hall, Inc., 1969), discusses relations among the disciplines, broad questions of utilization of the social sciences by society, and makes specific recommendations for public and university policy.

While close communication among all concerned has been the rule, the individual panel reports are the responsibility of the panels producing them. They have not been formally reviewed or approved by the Central Planning Committee or by the sponsoring organizations. They were reviewed at an earlier stage by representatives of the National Academy of Sciences and the Social Science Research Council.

Much of the data on the behavioral and social sciences in universities used in these reports comes from a 1968 questionnaire survey, conducted by the Survey Committee, of universities offering the PhD in one of these fields. Questionnaires were filled out by PhD-granting departments (referred to as the Departmental Questionnaire); by selected professional schools (referred to as the Professional School Questionnaire); by computation centers (referred to as the Computation Center Questionnaire); by university financial offices (referred to as the Administration Questionnaire); and by research institutes, centers, laboratories and museums engaged in research in the behavioral and social sciences (referred to as the Institute Questionnaire). Further information concerning this questionnaire survey is provided in the appendix to the general report of the Central Planning Committee, mentioned above.

Also included in the appendix of the report of the Central Planning Committee is a discussion of the method of degree projection used in these reports, as well as some alternative methods.

THE BEHAVIORAL AND SOCIAL SCIENCES SURVEY COMMITTEE
CENTRAL PLANNING COMMITTEE

Ernest R. Hilgard, *Stanford University*, CHAIRMAN
Henry W. Riecken, *Social Science Research Council*,
   Co-CHAIRMAN
Kenneth E. Clark, *University of Rochester*
James A. Davis, *Dartmouth College*
Fred R. Eggan, *The University of Chicago*
Heinz Eulau, *Stanford University*
Charles A. Ferguson, *Stanford University*
John L. Fischer, *Tulane University of Louisiana*
David A. Hamburg, *Stanford University*
Carl Kaysen, *Institute for Advanced Study*
William H. Kruskal, *The University of Chicago*
David S. Landes, *Harvard University*
James G. March, *University of California, Irvine*
George A. Miller, *The Rockefeller University*
Carl Pfaffmann, *The Rockefeller University*
Neil J. Smelser, *University of California, Berkeley*
Allan H. Smith, *Washington State University*
Robert M. Solow, *Massachusetts Institute of Technology*
Edward Taaffe, *The Ohio State University*
Charles Tilly, *The University of Michigan*
Stephen Viederman, *National Academy of Sciences*,
   EXECUTIVE OFFICER

ACKNOWLEDGMENTS

When the Psychiatry Panel was first organized, each member sent the chairman a set of background materials highly pertinent to the task at hand. With these vital resources in hand, the chairman prepared a first draft of the report.

It was my good fortune to be able to undertake this task during a fellowship year at the Center for Advanced Study in the Behavioral Sciences, Stanford, California. This is most appropriate, for the spirit of the Center pervades the report. Time and again, we have emphasized and illustrated the vital contributions of many disciplines. One of the main thrusts of the report is to promote contact, lively exchange, and mutual assistance among the various sciences concerned with man. This is precisely what the Center has stood for and done so much to implement. I take this occasion to express deep gratitude to the Center, not only for facilitating preparation of this report, but for its unique role in advancing the scientific study of behavior.

When the first draft was completed, feedback was obtained from many sources. The draft was reviewed not only by members of the Psychiatry Panel but by many others in psychiatry and related fields. I want especially to thank several persons who made an extraordinary contribution at this stage and were extremely helpful throughout: Drs. Albert J. Stunkard, Alberta E. Siegel, Jack Barchas, Eli Rubinstein, William Dement, and Beatrix Hamburg. In light of the extensive, constructive suggestions, the chairman prepared a second draft, which was reviewed by the Psychiatry Panel and by a special, inter-disciplinary panel appointed by the Committee of Science and Public Policy, National Academy of Sciences. These reviewers were Professors Julius Comroe, Daniel X. Freedman, Herbert McClosky, Robert S. Morison, and George Saslow. Their reviews were thorough and constructive, and we are indebted to them. When this review was completed, the chairman undertook a third and final version, which we now entrust to our readers. Before doing so, we want to thank Drs. Ernest Hilgard, Henry Riecken, and Stephen Viederman, who had the central responsibility for planning and guiding the entire series of survey reports on the behavioral and social sciences. They have done this difficult task with unfailing good judgment and, perhaps even more remarkable, good humor. In preparation of the psychiatry report, Mrs. Ann Morey cheerfully kept track of a mountain of papers and typed more versions than she cares to remember, for all of which we are grateful.

Finally, we must thank those who, perhaps more than any others, made this report possible—our patients. By trusting us and sharing their experiences with us and our colleagues throughout the field, they have provided the stimulus, sharpened the questions, and heightened our determination to find useful answers.

Many other persons were helpful to the Psychiatry Panel in preparation of this report. A few suggestions were sent anonymously, so we cannot thank their authors personally, but we are nevertheless grateful. From beginning to end, we have been impressed with the constructive and generous nature of the responses.

Mary Ainsworth, *Johns Hopkins University*
Bert Boothe, *National Institute of Mental Health*
John Paul Brady, *University of Pennsylvania*
Harvey Brooks, *Harvard University*
William Bunney, *National Institute of Mental Health*
George Coelho, *National Institute of Mental Health*
Preston Cutler, *Center for Advanced Study in the Behavioral Sciences*
Julian Davidson, *Stanford University*

Fred Elmadjian, *National Institute of Mental Health*
Solomon Goldberg, *National Institute of Mental Health*
Josephine Hilgard, *Stanford University*
Howard Hines, *National Science Foundation*
Harry Jerison, *Antioch College*
Eugene Kaplan, *National Naval Medical Center*
Herant Katchadourian, *Stanford University*
Seymour Kessler, *Stanford University*
Seymour Kety, *Harvard University*
William Kruskal, *University of Chicago*
Joshua Lederberg, *Stanford University*
Erich Lindemann, *Stanford University*
Lester Luborsky, *University of Pennsylvania*
Arnold Mandell, *University of California, San Diego*
Frederick Melges, *Stanford University*
Joe Mendels, *University of Pennsylvania*
Jack Mendelson, *National Institute of Mental Health*
Rudolf Moos, *Stanford University*
Donald Oken, *State University of New York, Upstate Medical Center*
Martin Orne, *University of Pennsylvania*
Betty Pickett, *National Institute of Mental Health*
William Pollin, *National Institute of Mental Health*
Merrill Read, *National Institute of Child Health and Human Development*
John Romano, *University of Rochester*
C. Peter Rosenbaum, *Stanford University*
Alan Rosenthal, *Stanford University*
Julius Segal, *National Institute of Mental Health*
Neil Smelser, *University of California, Berkeley*
Ralph Tyler, *Center for Advanced Study in the Behavioral Sciences*
Joan Warmbrunn, *Center for Advanced Study in the Behavioral Sciences*
Sherwood Washburn, *University of California, Berkeley*
Louis Wienckowski, *National Institute of Mental Health*

Meredith Wilson, *Center for Advanced Study in the Behavioral Sciences*
Paul Wilson, *American Psychiatric Association*
Lyman Wynne, *National Institute of Mental Health*
Eugene Yates, *University of Southern California*
Stanley Yolles, *National Institute of Mental Health*

CONTENTS

PSYCHIATRY AS A BEHAVIORAL SCIENCE

PREFACE

This book deals with the least-known aspects of psychiatry. Our task was part of a comprehensive survey of the behavioral sciences, and this report is one in a series of reports for the public on the whole range of scientific activities in the United States, initiated by the National Academy of Sciences and the Social Science Research Council. Therefore, we report here primarily on the *scientific* aspects of our field.

In order to make the scientific work meaningful, we have first sketched the scope and nature of psychiatric problems. What sorts of human suffering confront psychiatrists and their colleagues in closely related fields? Who cares for psychiatric patients now, and how? How did the field take its present form? And what clinical innovations are currently being tried to ease the burden of suffering and disability? These questions are considered in the first chapter. They give us some idea of the problems that need to be solved. The remainder of the book describes the various scientific ways of attempting their solution.

Some readers may be surprised by the variety of scientific approaches described in these chapters, and by the considerable emphasis on biological sciences. A word of explanation is in order. Scientific work on psychiatric problems is, for the most part, a recent development, and it is far less known and understood than the service aspects of the field. To a considerable extent, two images have dominated the public's view of psychiatry: the treatment of neurotic patients by privately practicing psychoanalysts, and the confinement

1

of psychotic patients to large, public mental hospitals. These are indeed two important facets of psychiatric activity, but in recent years the assortment of therapeutic activities has become much more varied, and the settings for scientific investigation of psychiatric problems have become quite different from traditional ones. So we here deliberately draw attention to the newest and least understood facets of the field.

This book depicts the biological sciences as emerging into full partnership with the better-known psychological and social approaches. There are several reasons for this emphasis. The biological sciences have lately produced developments of enormous significance —developments that have touched every aspect of living organisms. Especially in the past few years, much intellectual and technical effort has been directed toward understanding the brain and behavior. Scientists from backgrounds in physical and biological sciences, as well as those in behavioral sciences, have taken up the quest. This development is unprecedented in human history. No man can now know what the outcome of this unique effort will be; but there is growing evidence that the scientific community as a whole is becoming deeply concerned with human problems, and one focus of this concern lies in the area where psychiatrists have had much service responsibility.

Psychiatry's scientific position is at the interface between biological and behavioral sciences. In the universities, psychiatric scientists have benefited from contact with the new biology, and this contact has been considerably facilitated by the location of psychiatry departments in schools of medicine. This contact is much greater than that which most behavioral sciences have had with biology. At the same time, psychiatry has reached out more than any other medical specialty for contact with the emerging social sciences. Psychiatrists have learned from poignant experience that the human problems they face are too complex to be understood in any narrow, doctrinaire way. The tools of no single discipline will suffice. The present mood of the field is one that searches for new opportunities, welcomes diversity, and turns away from dogmatism.

Psychiatry is a highly visible field because it is concerned with so much suffering, and the wish for relief is so widespread. Much is expected of a profession assigned such important responsibilities by society—perhaps too much. The range of public attitudes toward the field is very great—from suspicion and even vituperation at one extreme to a romantic mystique of near-omniscience at the other. Psychiatry has been denounced by political extremists of the right and left. Yet, overall, public interest and respect have grown remarkably in recent decades. There has, for example, been much curiosity and puzzlement about certain prominent and controversial aspects of the field, especially psychoanalysis, drugs that affect brain and behavior, and comprehensive community mental health centers. Therefore, we have undertaken a state-of-the-art assessment in these areas. But for the most part we have looked ahead. We have taken some pains to indicate the limitations of present knowledge and to highlight the areas in which new help is needed. Above all, we have emphasized promising lines of inquiry and ways of mobilizing scientific strength more effectively for solutions of psychiatric problems. While we have indicated some satisfaction with the growth and accomplishments of this young field, we are much more interested in what psychiatry can *become*.

It was, of course, impossible to deal with all the subjects that deserved consideration. We have touched lightly on several topics that we would have preferred to discuss in detail. For example, the problem of drug abuse is now the subject of much attention. Unfortunately, its scientific investigation on any substantial scale is very recent. Still, we are beginning to see careful work on the abuse of various drugs, such as alcohol, opiates, barbiturates, amphetamines, and marijuana. These problems have recently become matters of intense public concern. The drugs are very widely employed with no medical supervision. The reasons for their widespread use touch on broad social questions, especially the problems of youth. It is difficult to get solid, dependable evidence on questions of drug use, but urgent efforts are being made to determine the effects of each drug at various dose levels in different kinds of persons. We need to know both short-term and long-term risks, the sought-after effects and the extent to which they are achieved, the personal characteristics and social settings most conducive to chronic drug use. Imaginative studies are being done on various treatment approaches, such as drug substitution, group therapy, and occupational preparation. Thus, a problem area that was socially neglected and virtually devoid of research a few years ago has come alive in response to an urgent need.

So it is with other problems. A generation ago, many psychiatrists believed that group therapy was no therapy at all. And for many years the area was clouded with undocumented claims. Only in the past few years have we begun to see a substantial body of carefully designed studies. Thus, research on group therapy might well have been considered here in more detail. The same may be said for many aspects of interpersonal relationships, which are, after all, at the center of most psychiatrists' professional interest and competence. For example, the research on development of close attachments between people, and the consequences of their disruption, might have been usefully considered at greater length. Similarly, we might well have discussed research on mental retardation; fortunately, this has been done in the general report, *The Behavioral and Social Sciences: Outlook and Needs* (Englewood Cliffs, N.J.: Prentice-Hall, 1969).

We express our regrets to the many fine clinicians and scientists whose work appears only briefly in these pages. A truly comprehensive assessment would have been far larger—and much more difficult to read. Our task here was to provide several *illustrative* lines of research in sufficient depth to convey the flavor of scientific work on psychiatric problems.

In this report, we have been primarily concerned with ways of *obtaining* new knowledge. We hope that others will consider ways of speeding the utilization of such knowledge as it becomes available. The day will come in this field, as it already has elsewhere, when the pace of advance is so rapid that effective utilization becomes difficult. Indeed, there is already a problem of sorting out insubstantial claims from dependable advances. Thus, the continuing education of psychiatrists, of nonpsychiatric physicians, and of the various mental health professionals, becomes increasingly important. No longer can we assume that a sound initial training meets all essential needs for a lifetime of professional work. Neither will the continuing, lifelong education of specialized professionals be adequate. The problems of human suffering which the public entrusts largely to psychiatry are too serious and too pervasive to remain in the specialized domain of any profession for long. They are matters on which an educated public in a democratic society demands to be informed. It is not surprising that newspapers, magazines, books, radio, and television are full of the problems of fear, hatred, despondency, and disintegration. The public has a direct and vital stake in objective assessment and effective utilization of research on psychiatric problems.

The series of survey reports on the behavioral sciences, of which this is one, has been broadly conceived in the service of an informed public. We have tried to write this book in such a way that its main features would be comprehensible and interesting to a wide range of thoughtful readers—making it as free of jargon as we were able. Nevertheless, we have felt it essential to face the difficulty and complexity inherent in the subject, and to give enough technical detail to provide accuracy and substance. We hope that it can be read with profit by persons in government, by students, by scientists in other fields, and indeed by anyone who wonders whether there is hope for solution of psychiatric problems.

1
A PERSPECTIVE ON PSYCHIATRY

THE FIELD OF PSYCHIATRY

To view psychiatry as a behavioral science is at once a paradox and an achievement. For psychiatry is not primarily a science, and until recently its links to science were quite tenuous. Psychiatry is a specialty within medicine, and although medicine is based in large part upon science, it is not itself a science. It is, instead, a profession, and its goals—the care of the sick and the relief of suffering—are different from those of science, which center on the search for knowledge.

Why then should psychiatry be represented in a survey of the behavioral sciences? Why should this occur at a time when there is an urgent need for fundamental, scientific understanding of human behavior? The answers to these questions may be found in the recent development of psychiatry, especially during the past three decades. During this period, psychiatry has concerned itself with many, diverse behavioral problems, and has achieved a measure of success in solving them. Even more important is the promise of some approaches pioneered by psychiatry in recent years, and the growing commitment of psychiatry (especially in the universities) to active participation in the behavioral science community.

This chapter describes the scope of psychiatry and the range of the problems to which it has addressed itself. The book then considers some of the approaches which have raised the hope that psychiatry may be able to contribute to the resolution of many of the problems facing our society today.

Psychiatry is a specialty within medicine. Psychiatrists hold the

7

MD degree. Further, specialized training is offered in medical centers to physicians who serve as residents in psychiatry for a three-year period. Most medical students enter a residency immediately after attaining the MD and completing a year's internship at an accredited hospital; but some enter a psychiatry residency after an intervening period of military service, medical practice, research, or work in another medical specialty.

Since we are concerned here with psychiatry as a behavioral science, we will omit or minimize many topics that might be central to a discussion of psychiatry as a medical specialty. For example, ethical problems arising during psychiatric treatment are a vital concern in the field, but we discuss them only as they bear on behavioral science research by psychiatrists. There are several such topics which we have ignored or mentioned only cursorily, in order to highlight those topics within psychiatry which bear most directly on the domain of the behavioral sciences.

RECENT HISTORICAL BACKGROUND

Until recently, it was possible to define psychiatry and to delimit its scope with a measure of precision and considerable general agreement. For years psychiatry has been "that branch of medicine which deals with the diagnosis, prevention, and treatment of mental illness." There was general agreement that "mental illness" consisted of disturbed behavior, usually of such severity as to require hospitalization of the patient for his own safety or the safety of others. Today the field is growing and changing so rapidly that even its leaders are uncertain about its scope.

It is frequently said that mental illness is the leading health problem in America today. Figures on its prevalence confirm this statement. During the past decade, nearly 40 percent of all hospital beds in the United States were occupied by the mentally ill, with about half a million patients hospitalized in psychiatric facilities at any given time. During the coming year, about one million Americans will become disturbed enough to require psychiatric hospitalization. It has been estimated that 2 percent of persons born this year will at some time during their lives suffer from schizophrenia, the most severe of the mental illnesses (described in greater detail later in this report) and, under certain circumstances, this proportion could go as high as 6 percent. The best current estimates indicate that one American out of twelve will require psychiatric hospitalization at some time during the course of his life, and almost everyone will have experience with severe mental illness in a close friend or relative.

Formidable as they are, these figures almost certainly understate the extent of the problem. They are based upon hospital admission statistics, and take no account of the number of persons suffering from mental illness who are never admitted to a hospital. Information about these sufferers can be obtained only by the difficult and expensive method of careful house-to-house surveys, and few such surveys have ever been made. The surveys that have been conducted suggest that the number of mentally ill persons who have not received treatment well may exceed the number who are treated. Two of the most careful surveys estimate that between 10 and 24 percent of the population may suffer from "mental disorder" or be "seriously impaired by mental disorder."

To psychiatry's traditional concern with the diagnosis and treatment of mental illness has been added a wide range of new problems and new tasks, some already accepted as medical, others from outside the traditional medical domain. In light of such rapid growth and change, it may be useful to review the scope of psychiatry from a historical point of view.

Psychiatry is dependent upon the social climate in which it exists, a dependence that becomes critical during periods of growth and development. This feature of psychiatry is unusual among the specialties of medicine. In general, psychiatry flourishes during periods characterized by an emphasis upon political freedom, personal liberty, concern with the development of human potential, and belief in the possibilities for improvement of man. By contrast, the field fares poorly during periods of political repression, infringement of personal liberty, and pessimistic assumptions regarding the nature of man. It may well be that the encouraging achievements of American psychiatry are in part a product of a climate of values that facilitates the study of man and believes in the possibilities for human improvement.

These social considerations appear to have been of determining importance during the period, nearly two hundred years ago, when psychiatry was established. Influenced by the ideals of the French Revolution, and by those of Quaker hospital reform, physicians in France and England took the momentous step of selecting for special treatment, from a variety of the socially disabled, those persons suffering from mental illness. They defined a diagnosis of severe mental illness and instituted nonpunitive care. Special hospitals were established to offer care to this newly defined group of patients. By their demonstration of the effectiveness of a uniquely humane concern for these patients—by their so-called "moral treatment of the insane"—these pioneers laid the groundwork for modern psychiatry.

The second phase of development in American psychiatry was heralded by World War II. The heightened concern with political freedom and personal liberty was probably a catalyst for change. Another factor certainly was the wartime experience with psychiatric disability, both at the induction centers and on the battlefields. Nothing in our experience had prepared us for the shockingly high rates of psychiatric disability found among presumably healthy young men. The number of Americans classified as unfit for military service for neuropsychiatric reasons was 1,846,000, well over 10 percent of all registrants examined. Of the men who passed this screening and went on to military service, about one million, or nearly 10 percent, were hospitalized for neurophychiatric reasons, and about 500,000 received psychiatric discharges from the service. Clearly, psychiatric disturbance was a far more widespread problem than had ever before been recognized.

Most of these disabilities were neurotic rather than psychotic. The men had emotional disorders entailing much suffering, personal ineffectiveness, and wasted potential, but not severe enough to require prolonged hospitalization. A strong demand for treatment of such disturbances began to emerge.

This demand came at a critical juncture in the development of American psychiatry, a period in which the ideas and principles of psychoanalysis were being introduced into the country by psychoanalysts who had fled Nazi persecution during the 1930s. Just at this period when society demanded of the medical profession a concern with neurosis, psychoanalysis made available to psychiatrists, for the first time, a systematic theory of neurosis and a therapy which held promise for its cure. There was, further, the inspiring example of many psychoanalysts, with their detailed attention to motivation and emotion, their concern with effects of early experience upon later behavior, and their sustained therapeutic interest in their neurotic patients.

It would be hard to overestimate the impact upon American psychiatry of this interaction of social need and psychoanalysis. Within a few years, it shattered the long-standing pessimism born of years of heartbreak in the treatment of the psychoses, and it imbued American psychiatry with enthusiasm. It brought neurosis out of the limbo of public and medical disdain, eliciting new interest and hope. Indeed, patterns of medical education, practice, and research were altered to encompass emotional disturbances. For a decade following World War II, psychoanalysis was clearly the dominant force in American psychiatry, and it continues to exert strong influence to-day. For these reasons, we wish to provide some brief perspective on psychoanalysis, especially its impact on psychiatry as a behavioral science.

Psychoanalysis has three major facets: a body of observations, concepts and hypotheses, a technique of therapy and research, and a profession. Freud, the founder of psychoanalysis, was a highly independent, creative, and courageous scholar. He made novel observations and suggested unconventional and provocative hypotheses. He was keenly interested in the biological and social sciences of his day. These wide interests are reflected throughout the body of his writing. Thus, psychoanalysis began with independent-minded, searching observation and broad scholarship. However, Freud and his early followers met with harsh criticism, ridicule, and even ostracism. During its most formative years, the psychoanalytic movement was largely cut off from the universities. Only in America, and after many years, was there a broadly enthusiastic response.

The initially hostile reception to psychoanalytic innovation probably contributed to a defender-of-the-faith orientation in some psychoanalytic professional organizations. In any event, it now seems clear that the period of psychoanalytic innovation was followed by a period of psychoanalytic conservatism in which further innovation was not encouraged. In many fields of inquiry, after an initial creative period, there is often a tendency for followers to identify with the founder's specific set of beliefs rather than with his spirit of discovery. What starts as a constructive reform, therefore, becomes resistant to change, and an organization forms to protect the discoveries of the admired innovator. Psychoanalysis went through a period of this sort, but recently it has been liberalized and brought into contact with other disciplines, especially in the universities.

The psychoanalytic body of observations, concepts, and hypotheses has had a strong influence on psychiatry and related fields in the

United States. Psychoanalysis offered powerful suggestions, in an ambitious and sweeping effort to explain much of human suffering. After a half-century's experience, we can now say with reasonable accuracy that the hopes and expectations aroused by these psychoanalytic suggestions were excessive. Moreover, the therapeutic limitations of psychoanalytic treatment were underestimated in some respects, even though Freud had carefully called attention to them. Nonetheless, psychoanalytic thought has had a stimulating effect on the development of the behavioral sciences, while psychoanalytic treatment has awakened interest in psychotherapeutic approaches to a wide range of problems—indeed, much wider than Freud envisioned. One need not adhere to any rigid, doctrinaire view of psychoanalysis to appreciate its stimulating impact on many facets of American psychiatry. Although in the future psychoanalytic thinking will no longer dominate American psychiatry, it will continue to be important—one among many approaches in a complex, diversified, pluralistic area of human endeavor.

During World War II a great number of Americans were exposed to vivid experiences of psychological stress—separation, loss, bereavement, injury, death, and personal dislocations of many kinds. Experiences of intense emotional distress, personal disorganization, and "nervous breakdown" were common. Although often the symptoms were very alarming, rapid recovery usually occurred, and psychiatrists were able to be useful in aiding recovery. This was encouraging to psychiatrists and enhanced the progress of their field. During and shortly after the war, the mass media publicized the many heartening recoveries. In this context, too, psychoanalytic ideas attracted much attention. By the late 1940s, public interest in the origins and possible cure of behavior disorders was widespread and optimistic. This interest supported a number of significant developments in the postwar years—explosive growth of psychiatric training programs in medical schools and teaching hospitals; a rapid expansion of outpatient psychotherapy, mainly based on psychoanalytic concepts and financed on a private, fee-for-service basis; formation of psychiatric units in general hospitals, where very few had existed before; and progressive federal government programs broadly supporting research, education, and service in the field of mental health. These developments were promising and exciting. From the widening circles of hope, many talented workers were drawn into the mental health professions.

Yet some important areas were neglected. In their enthusiasm for psychoanalysis, some psychiatrists ignored other sources of new information. Little psychiatric attention was given to some of the severe disorders that constitute serious social problems, such as mental retardation, alcoholism, and suicidal depression. There was no financial mechanism to support psychiatric concern for population groups with low economic status, including those with future economic potential but current low income, such as college students. The main thrust of the postwar efforts was toward disorders of moderate severity in the affluent sector of society. The public mental hospitals, dealing with more severe and protracted problems, were not at first greatly affected, but they changed markedly in the mid-1950s, as we shall see. Research, too, was not rapidly affected. Indeed, it is only in the past decade that a sizeable cadre of well-trained scientists has emerged in psychiatry.

A significant new phase in American psychiatry began in 1955. In that year, responding to growing demands for improvement in the care of the mentally ill, the American Psychiatric Association took the initiative in persuading Congress to appropriate funds for a Joint Commission on Mental Health and Illness. While the Joint Commission was conducting its deliberations, the effectiveness of new drugs for the treatment of severe mental illness was being established by research in the U.S. and in other countries. These drugs accelerated the shift of mental hospitals from custodial to therapeutic activity, which had begun earlier under the impetus of psychotherapeutic and sociotherapeutic efforts. Because these drugs were available, many patients who would otherwise have been confined to hospitals could be treated in their home communities and continue to live at home. In this hopeful context, the Joint Commission presented its report to the Congress in 1961. President Kennedy promptly appointed an interagency task force to make recommendations for its implementation. When this task was done, he presented to the Congress in 1963 his Special Message on Mental Illness and Mental Retardation, the first of its kind by an American president. In speaking of the suffering of the mentally ill and the mentally retarded and of their families, he said

> This situation has been tolerated far too long. It has troubled our national conscience, but only as a problem unpleasant to mention, easy to postpone and despairing of solution. The Federal Government, despite the na-

tional impact of the problem, has largely left the problem up to the States. The States have depended on custodial hospitals and homes. Many such hospitals and homes have been shamefully understaffed, overcrowded institutions from which death too often provided the only firm hope of release. The time has come for a bold new approach. New medical, scientific, and social tools and insights are now available.

Soon afterwards, the Congress passed the Community Mental Health Centers Act of 1963 and, with President Johnson's sponsorship, its 1965 extension to provide funds to staff these centers. The Act aims to provide for all segments of society the kind of prompt, comprehensive, and continuous mental health services that have been available until recently only to the wealthy. For this purpose, community mental health centers are being established in the heart of the geographic areas they will serve, each designed to fit the special needs and assets of the people in its area. In order to provide the greatest possible flexibility of treatment, each center must contain certain essential elements—inpatient hospital facilities, an outpatient clinic, transitional facilities (such as day hospitals, night hospitals, and half-way houses), emergency services, and services for education and consultation on mental health problems throughout the community. The implementation of this promising program has proceeded rapidly from its modest beginning in 1965. By the end of 1969, 210 comprehensive community mental health services were operational, serving a population of 29 million people. In another decade, about 1000 centers should be making care available to everyone in the country.

The major purpose of this plan is to make mental health services available quickly and at reasonable cost to anyone who needs such help. It is to be provided locally, by well-qualified professionals, and in a manner that avoids stigma. It aims to replace a system in which the mentally ill are neglected in huge, isolated human warehouses far from family, friends, and voluntary help. Considering the ambitious goals of these comprehensive community health centers, what is the range of relevant information and skills they will draw upon? Surely the range is very broad. It is not confined to a subdivision of psychiatry, called community psychiatry, though such a subspecialty may provide some of the leadership. The range of information and skills that will be required in these centers cuts very broadly through biological and behavioral sciences, as well as across the several mental health professions. Much research will be necessary to provide means to achieve the goal of community mental health.

The community mental health center program is a part of a larger social movement—what has often been called the revolution of rising expectations. This revolution is one of rising expectations of health services. Like most social movements, this one is presently based on quite limited information. It is not entirely an application of scientific principles, though it is partially so. This social current emerges from humanitarian values, as did the very beginning of psychiatry two hundred years ago. It may well provide a major stimulus for the development of relevant supporting sciences.

The receptive social climate and the generous public support for psychiatry today have, as in past periods of development of the field, been met by new therapeutic instruments and theories. This time, however, instead of needing to rely on a single theoretical and therapeutic approach, as when psychoanalysis made its great contribution to American psychiatry, we have several on which we can draw. These can be divided, somewhat arbitrarily, into those that have developed out of clinical practice, and those that represent the application of knowledge from the basic sciences.

Psychoanalysis, of course, continues to be one of the major psychotherapeutic approaches. Efforts to make it applicable to a larger number of patients, suffering from a wide range of disorders, have led to the development of new techniques of individual psychotherapy. In addition, the requirements and opportunities of treating large numbers of patients have stimulated the development of group therapy. One special form of group therapy involves a family rather than an individual as the treatment unit. As psychiatrists continue in the tradition of concern for hospital treatment of the mentally ill, increasingly sophisticated formulations about therapeutic properties of the hospital environment have led to a form of treatment called milieu therapy.

It would be difficult to overestimate the importance of the many contributions of the basic sciences to the understanding and treatment of mental illness. We will mention only two of the most important ones. The first is the development of drugs for the treatment of mental illness. Drugs effective in the treatment of schizophrenia became available over a decade ago. More recently we have had a growing number of agents for the relief of emotional distress. Currently, there is hope that new agents are effective with depression. These will be discussed in some detail in a later section of this report. The second important contribution is the development of behavioral therapies that apply principles of learning elucidated in psychology laboratories. From an initial concern with mild and then more severe neurotic fears and inhibitions, these therapies have now been used in the care of severely disturbed patients in mental hospitals, the treatment of delinquent behavior, alcoholism, and the socialization of the mentally retarded.

One of the strongest influences in psychiatry today is its growing concern not only for the individual patient but also for the mental health of the population as a whole. A growing social orientation was markedly accelerated by the Community Mental Health Centers Act. This expansion, in perspective, has drawn greater attention to the social environment, to the coordination of patient care services, and to the eventual prevention of mental disorders. The boundaries of the field in these areas of newer concern are unclear, and there is considerable disagreement among psychiatrists about the definition of our expanded domain of responsibility.

SCOPE OF PSYCHIATRIC TASKS

Although the very new tasks of psychiatry may receive more publicity, the greatest progress has probably been made in the established areas. The Community Mental Health Centers Act has stimulated considerable growth in the facilities available for the treatment of persons suffering from psychoses and neuroses. Of the many possible illustrations we will mention only two: the growth of outpatient clinics and the growth of psychiatric units in general hospitals. Both types of institutions are of the greatest importance in providing alternatives to confinement in what are often merely custodial institutions. Both furnish readily available treatment with minimal social stigma, and both help keep patients close to their families and communities during brief episodes of emotional disturbance. Indeed, in its focus on prompt treatment and on care in the community, the community mental health center concept draws heavily on the experience of outpatient clinics and psychiatric units in general hospitals. Such facilities are vital features of the newly established community mental health centers.

Table 1-1 shows the remarkable growth of psychiatric outpatient clinics during the past thirty-seven years. During the past year, well over one million persons were treated in such clinics; no doubt this saved some from the occurrence of more severe mental illness, relieved neurotic problems in others, and helped to rehabilitate still others who had been discharged from mental hospitals.

TABLE 1-1 GROWTH OF PSYCHIATRIC OUTPATIENT CLINICS IN THE UNITED STATES

Year	Number
1930	217
1940	372
1950	783
1960	1502
(1967)	2259

Source: National Institute of Mental Health

The growth of psychiatric units in general hospitals has been even more rapid. Prior to World War II, there were only 37 such units in the entire country, and nowhere was the isolation of psychiatry from American medicine more poignantly demonstrated than in the exclusion of psychiatric patients from general hospitals. This situation changed radically when wartime experience showed that psychiatric units could be incorporated into military general hospitals, and that psychiatric treatment in this setting could be effective. By 1946, 109 general hospitals had established psychiatric units, and by 1968 over 1000 such units were in operation. Although such units tend to be small, they have had an influence out of all proportion to their size. In the last year for which such figures are available, for example, the 36,000 beds in psychiatric units in general hospitals admitted more patients than did the 660,000 beds in all other psychiatric facilities combined! Table 1-2 shows the extent of this extraordinary phenomenon.

Public mental hospitals have also been changing remarkably since World War II. This change is based on humanitarian values and

TABLE 1-2   HOSPITAL ADMISSIONS TO PSYCHIATRIC FACILITIES IN THE UNITED STATES

Facility	1963	1966
Psychiatric units in general hospitals	212,000	446,000
All other psychiatric facilities	283,000	327,000

Source: National Institute of Mental Health

has been assisted substantially by the advent of the newer drug therapies. The emphasis on therapy as well as custody and protection has led to efforts to restore the dignity of the mentally ill person, to enhance his feeling of personal worth, and to establish relations with him on the basis of mutual respect.

The modern mental hospital is designed to be a therapeutic community. It aims to minimize the punitive features of older prison-like facilities. To the greatest extent possible, active treatment replaces custody. Typically, wards are unlocked, patients have freedom of movement, and staff members participate with patients in group activities, though privacy is also preserved. The patient's individuality is emphasized. It has become clear that patient groups are capable of handling considerable responsibility. Increasingly, they have been given a voice in determining the conditions of their lives in the hospital. Efforts have been made to increase their association with family and friends. Volunteers, including many college students, have come into the hospital. Many large public mental hospitals have introduced a unit system in which the hospital is divided into smaller components, each responsible for a geographic region. This helps to maintain ties with the patient's home community and to improve the patient's circumstances upon his return. Altogether, the old atmosphere of lethargy and pessimism has given way to a sense of movement and a newer climate of expectation envisioning recovery.

A major development of the past two decades has been the emergence of transitional facilities that serve as bridges between full-time hospitalization and independent community living. These transitional facilities include partial hospitalization and community treatment services. The best known of these are the *day hospital*, for patients who are able to return to their own homes at night; the *night hospital*, which enables patients to continue their normal daily activities (usually employment) but provides a protected situation for the night hours; the *halfway house*, a residence for formerly hospitalized individuals, combined with aftercare (posthospital) services; *family care* or foster placement, with the patient assigned to live in a family's home; and admission screening and home treatment services. All are products of a search for effective alternatives to chronic hospitalization.

Child psychiatry has been a recognized activity for the past fifty years, and the child guidance movement gave rise to hopes that treatment of the emotional disorders of childhood might prevent the development of more serious illness in adult life. While these hopes have not yet been fulfilled, there is now a burst of new activity, including family therapy, consultation within the school, and direct action to alter and improve the social environments in which children grow up.

Forensic psychiatry is another subspecialty with a long history, particularly of court testimony by psychiatrists on the competence of the accused to face trial and to conduct personal affairs. Such relatively unpromising and often poorly regarded activities are now being supplemented by serious collaboration between psychiatrists and lawyers on fundamental legal problems. A growing number of psychiatrists are becoming involved in the treatment and study of persons confined in prisons, in efforts at rehabilitation of offenders, and in research on criminal behavior and its prevention.

Military psychiatry, which received an enormous impetus from the disturbing revelations of World War II, has continued to increase in effectiveness during the subsequent years. A high proportion of relatively unstable inductees have been salvaged for military service, and the huge psychiatric rejection rates characteristic of the early periods of World War II have been markedly reduced. Furthermore, psychiatric disability arising in both combat and noncombatant duty has been steadily reduced, and ingenious treatment techniques for those servicemen who do break down have been so effective that they have in some instances been adopted for civilian use.

Mental retardation has long been one of the most neglected handicaps in our society, and even today we have only begun to provide the kind of care which may bring dignity and a measure of personal effectiveness to the mentally retarded. The problem has dimensions far beyond the purview of psychiatry, involving such other medical specialties as pediatrics and neurology, along with education, psychology, social work, and vocational rehabilitation. Nevertheless, psychiatrists can make important contributions to the care of the mentally retarded, and a growing number of psychiatrists are concerning themselves with this problem.

Alcoholism and drug addiction have been public health problems in this country for many years, and even the rough estimates now available make clear their terrible cost. Consider alcoholism. From four to five million Americans suffer from chronic alcoholism, and at least 11,000 deaths per year are caused by this condition. The indirect costs are far higher. For example, it is estimated that alcohol is implicated in more than half of all motor vehicle accidents. This fact gains in impressiveness when we note that the National Safety Council has reported that traffic accidents in 1965 took 49,000 lives and caused 1,800,000 disabling injuries. The cost of alcoholism to industry has been estimated to exceed two billion dollars a year.

Psychiatry has shared in the traditional apathy and indifference of the medical profession to alcoholism, even though certain dedicated psychiatrists have been leaders in the few efforts to control alcoholism and drug addiction. Within the past two years, however, the National Institute of Mental Health has established a National Center for the Prevention and Control of Alcoholism and a Center for Studies of Narcotic and Drug Abuse. These twin centers have embarked on ambitious programs of research and treatment. Similarly, the Veterans Administration has recently undertaken a program of research on problems of alcohol. These progressive steps remind us how new is our effort to achieve practical understanding of addiction.

Aging has long been an involuntary concern of psychiatry, because of the institutionalization in mental hospitals of those aged persons who could no longer be maintained in the community. But it was a concern that had aroused little direct action, and only the very high death rates of the aged shortly after hospitalization (as high as 50 percent during the first six months) prevented the aged from occupying a far more prominent place in our mental hospitals. Again, the problem has dimensions that extend beyond psychiatry. But psychiatrists have begun to direct their attention to it with programs of research and education that give promise of more humane care for the aged. We note with encouragement the growing development of facilities specifically designed for the aged.

Industrial psychiatry was one of the earliest psychiatric disciplines to exploit the use of the consultant's role, and to indicate what can be achieved not only by direct patient care but also by indirect consultation to modify harmful factors in the social environment. Demand for such services has continued to grow, from management and labor alike. There has been a very rapid recent growth in mental health programs sponsored by some of the most prominent labor unions.

Suicide is now the tenth ranking cause of death in the United States, and more accurate reporting might well accord it a higher rank. It is a particularly serious problem among certain groups—the elderly, college students and other college-age persons (among whom suicide is actually the third ranking cause of death), the jobless, and depreciated minority groups. Despite the extent of this problem, until recently there has been little systematic research, therapeutic innovation, and preventive effort directed toward suicide. Three years ago the National Institute of Mental Health established a Center for Studies of Suicide Prevention. This Center has embarked on a research program into the causes of suicide and the means for its prevention. It has established an interdisciplinary university-based research and training center. And it has provided support for the development of community-based Suicide Prevention Centers, whose widely publicized telephone numbers may be used to obtain immediate help at any time by a person contemplating suicide.

Problems of poverty have long been an indirect concern of psychiatry. Poor people entered the mental hospitals and stayed there with a frequency out of all proportion to their numbers in the general population. In part, this occurred because of the inadequate resources for reintegrating them into their home communities. Until very recently, psychiatrists had confined their efforts to treating the social casualties as they were brought in off the battlefields of the slums and ghettos, and had little hope of intervening effectively at the site where the casualties were occurring. Today, psychiatrists are working among the poor, searching for ways to understand and alleviate the social influences on mental illness. One interesting innovation has been the establishment of storefront clinics, situated in areas of extreme poverty, which provide service to persons who would be very unlikely to utilize conventional psychiatric facilities. Necessity forces psychiatrists in the storefront clinics to deal with such personal and social problems as job opportunities, unemployment compensation, welfare checks, slum housing, and the aura of helplessness and suspicion which lies over the slums.

THE RECORD OF ACHIEVEMENT

We have discussed the scope of psychiatry and the expansion of responsibilities it has undertaken in recent years. We have not, however, documented the effectiveness of its activities; indeed, their effectiveness has not been adequately assessed. Yet if society charges a profession with the stewardship of some of its major problems, that profession must have achieved more than the mere proliferation of services. What is the record?

We cannot undertake here a comprehensive account of the effectiveness of even those relatively few psychiatric programs that have been evaluated. The oldest concern of psychiatry is with overt mental illness, particularly with those persons whose behavior is so disturbed as to require hospitalization. What have been the results of this concern? The record of the treatment of severe mental illness has taken a heartening turn in recent years. Figure 1-1 gives a graphic account of the changing number of patients in state and county mental hospitals. These institutions account for the vast majority of patients hospitalized for mental illness. For many years, this number had been increasing at an average annual rate of over 2 percent. Although improved treatment had, in recent years, begun to return more and more patients to the community, until 1956 the number of patients released from hospitals was not sufficiently high to offset the rise in number admitted, and the mental hospital population continued to grow.

A historical turning point occurred at the end of 1955, when the patient population reached its peak of 559,000. The following year, for the first time, the number of patients in mental hospitals did not increase, and, in fact, declined. This decline has continued for each of the succeeding years, and its rate has accelerated. This decline is all the more remarkable when one considers that most public mental hospitals are grossly understaffed.

By the end of 1967, the patient population had fallen to 426,000; and by mid-June of 1968 to 401,000. These decreases occurred despite the continuing rapid increase in the population at large. Figure 1-1

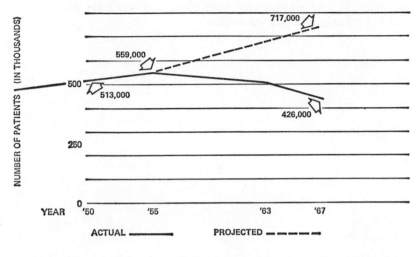

PROJECTED AND ACTUAL NUMBERS OF RESIDENT PATIENTS

END OF YEAR, STATE AND COUNTY MENTAL HOSPITALS 1946 - 1973

FIGURE 1-1

shows the real magnitude of the achievement in reducing the number of hospitalized mentally ill from the 1955 peak of 559,000. Had the earlier trend continued, the number in mental hospitals would now be about 717,000. Part of this success can be attributed to the effectiveness with which psychiatry has managed its traditional task. We are not suggesting that these discharged patients are free of difficulty. Many continue in treatment in outpatient and transitional facilities. The fact remains that, under these new conditions, they are more likely to maintain family ties, be productive economically, and participate in community life. (For additional research on assessment of treatment effectiveness, see the sections, Psychopharmacology and Psychotherapy in Chapter 3.)

In the chapters that follow, we consider first some of the common disorders with which psychiatry is concerned—schizophrenia, depression, and disorders of childhood—and some new ways of understanding them. We then discuss two areas in which new methods are being developed to provide more effective treatment than was available in former years—drug treatment and psychotherapy. There follows a discussion of representative areas of research in which psychiatrists have played an important part, and of some investigations that have transformed our ways of thinking about certain psychiatric problems. Finally, we consider some plans and hopes for the development of psychiatry in the years ahead.

2
RESEARCH ON PSYCHIATRIC DISORDERS

SCHIZOPHRENIA

Schizophrenia, the most common form of psychosis, is one of the world's most important health problems. Schizophrenia is a profound behavior disorder, typically characterized by gross distortions of reality, including delusions and hallucinations. Speech and mannerisms are often bizarre. Frequently the emotions expressed are entirely inappropriate to the thoughts and actions of the patient. There is profound and pervasive distrust of other people and extreme withdrawal from close human relations. The risk of harm to self or others is unusually high in schizophrenia as compared to other forms of mental illness. About one-fourth of the patients admitted each year to public mental hospitals are diagnosed as suffering schizophrenic reactions; about half the resident population of all hospitals are schizophrenics. Economically, the high cost of schizophrenia arises from the fact that the disease has its greatest impact during the most productive years of life. Three-fourths of all first-admission schizophrenics are between fifteen and forty-four years of age; the median age is thirty-three years.

Scientific investigation of schizophrenia has encountered many pitfalls. As elsewhere in psychiatry, the intense human suffering involved has provided a stimulus for wishful thinking. The "cause" and "cure" of schizophrenia have been "discovered" many times, but we are still in the dark. Let us briefly sketch some of the newer scientific approaches in investigating this problem. It should be emphasized that the research reported here is not viewed as providing definitive answers. Rather, we have selected certain lines of inquiry that illustrate

25

a sense of constructive movement in the problem area. Other lines of inquiry might equally well have been reported. It is not possible in this report to describe all promising research efforts on psychiatric problems. The criteria we have used in selecting our examples in this section and elsewhere are: (1) involvement of scientists from several disciplines; (2) formulation of important research questions; and (3) a momentum in research activity likely to yield valuable information even if currently attractive hypotheses fail to be proven. We will begin with biological approaches and then consider psychological and social research.

In the neurophysiological sphere, advances in instrumentation, especially in computer applications, have improved measurement of the brain's electrical activity in schizophrenia and other conditions. Such studies can now be performed through the intact scalp and yield more precise and reliable information than the traditional electroencephalogram (EEG). These techniques are capable of demonstrating significant differences between psychotic patients and normal controls, but it is not yet known whether any of them are specific to schizophrenia. Similar investigations are being conducted in depressive conditions. These techniques, such as the averaged evoked potential in response to specific sensory stimulation, are also being used to measure effects of drugs and hormones on brain function.

In the biochemical sphere, research has centered upon two approaches—abnormality of neuroregulatory agents, and abnormality of blood proteins. The term neuroregulatory agents refers to a variety of chemical compounds that may function as transmitters between nerve cells at synapses or as modulators of neural function within cells, or between nerve cells and glial cells in the brain. Examples are the catecholamines (noradrenalin, dopamine, and adrenalin) and the indoleamines (such as serotonin). Interest in these compounds has been stimulated by finding that many drugs which profoundly affect behavior also affect metabolism of neuroregulatory agents. Further, some derivatives of these compounds are capable of producing hallucinations. If such compounds are transmitters, there are a number of ways in which influences upon them could affect behavior. Susceptible processes could include formation, storage, release, metabolic disposition and re-uptake, or interaction with receptors. Any of these processes might be influenced by genetic and/or stress variables. It is now known that stress affects these compounds in brain.

One approach under active investigation in a number of laboratories involves the search for abnormal metabolites of neuroregulatory agents. Examples of this line of inquiry will now be cited.

A psychiatric-biochemical research team suggested an interesting hypothesis many years ago that led to much subsequent research. They proposed that transmethylation, the adding of a methyl group, was an important process in the metabolism of catecholamines— chemical compounds of the type exemplified by the well-known adrenalin and its close relative, noradrenalin. This prediction was confirmed a decade later in basic research on catecholamine metabolism. Several methylated derivatives of catecholamines (such as mescaline) produce symptoms similar to those of schizophrenic psychosis. This raises the question of whether some abnormal metabolite of the catecholamines, particularly a methylated metabolite, might produce symptoms of schizophrenia, especially under stress, when catecholamines are secreted in large amounts. This hypothesis was tested by giving large doses of methionine (a methyl donor) to some chronic schizophrenics, who had agreed to participate, and by giving an inhibitor which would prevent the normal destruction of amines. Thus, the experimental conditions favored the accumulation of methylated amines and might be expected to cause a temporary flareup in the patients' characteristic schizophrenic symptoms. About one-third of the patients did indeed react with a marked intensification of their symptoms. However, it is not definitively established whether the investigators have merely imposed a new, transient toxic psychosis in a schizophrenic patient, analogous to an alcoholic binge. This is an example of the difficulties in biochemical research on severe mental disorders. The fact that methionine does intensify psychosis in some patients has been confirmed by several groups. Betaine, another methyl donor, gives similar results. Amino acids that are not methyl donors have not given results of this sort. Hence, there is now considerable interest in the possibility that a methylation process has gone awry in schizophrenia.

A related line of inquiry has elicited much interest recently. It began with a report that dimethoxyphenylethylamine (DMPEA or "pink spot") is present in the urine of schizophrenic patients. Since this compound is very similar to the hallucinogenic drug, mescaline, the finding if confirmed would suggest that these unfortunate persons were producing an internal toxic substance that adversely affected brain function. Laboratories in several countries have joined this search, but results have so far been equivocal. One of the best of these studies took the precaution of having the examination of patients and urine done independently and "blind." (That is, each examiner had no information on other measures, thus eliminating observer bias.) When the data were decoded, the results clearly demonstrated that in the patients who were definitely schizophrenic there was a high percentage in whom the pink spot was found. In patients who were questionably schizophrenic, a lower but still significant number showed urinary pink spots. In patients who were not schizophrenic, the urine examination was negative, with only one exception. Yet a serious difficulty remains: the investigators did not control drug administration. The metabolites of the phenothiazines (the major tranquilizers) continue to appear in a patient's urine for weeks after he has stopped taking the tranquilizer. They can cause a variety of colored spots in chromatograms of urine. Since schizophrenic patients nowadays are almost always treated with such drugs, this presents a serious problem in interpreting the results. Again, it is a typical problem in studying severe mental disorder. In any event, more refined methods are now being used in an effort to characterize chemically the urinary pink spot, particularly whether it is invariably DMPEA. If this should be established, its causal relation to a subgroup of schizophrenic patients would then require investigation.

Another hypothesis in this field, similar in nature and origin, is interesting because it illustrates the stimulating effect of a clinical problem upon basic research. Some years ago the suggestion was made that schizophrenia might be produced by abnormal metabolism of adrenalin, such that a hallucinogenic compound would be produced internally. Adrenochrome was proposed as the most likely causal agent. Since virtually nothing was known of the normal metabolism of adrenalin, let alone its metabolism in schizophrenia, this hypothesis remained untested for some years. Then it was taken up by an interdisciplinary group, including both clinical and basic investigators. They recognized that the radiolabeled adrenalin then available did not contain large enough amounts of radioactivity. Adrenalin is so potent, and a safe dose is so small, that a very high degree of radiolabeling is required to carry out meaningful studies on its metabolic fate. This requirement was met, and the research group quickly worked out the metabolism of adrenalin. Today, over 95 percent of its metabolic products can be accounted for, and this basic information made it possible to examine the metabolism of labeled adrenalin in schizophrenics. When this was done, schizophrenics showed essentially the same patterns of metabolites from peripherally administered adrenalin as did normal persons. No evidence of abnormal metabolites was found. However, the basic knowledge of adrenalin metabolism achieved by this and related investigations on the metabolism of amines has proven to be of great value in clarifying the important role of catecholamines in the brain and throughout the body. This knowledge is likely to be important in understanding a variety of diseases (such as hypertension and depressions), whatever its ultimate significance for schizophrenia.

Not only have catecholamines been investigated, but the indoleamines, such as serotonin, have also been the subject of research. Metabolites of serotonin, such as bufotenine, are being investigated in a number of laboratories to determine whether any of them can be found in body tissues of patients with various types of mental illness. In addition, investigators with an interest in organic chemistry are trying to determine the structure-activity relation between some of the hallucinogenic agents and agents found naturally in the brain. No direct relationship to schizophrenia has yet been demonstrated. However, as with the catecholamines, the discoveries about indoleamine metabolism that have already emerged have proven to be of value in clarifying important roles of these compounds in the brain and throughout the body.

The second major line of inquiry in the biochemical sphere concerns possible protein abnormalities in the blood of schizophrenics. Research efforts in the past decade have been persistent but inconclusive in this area. Recently, investigators have suggested that a protein in the blood of schizophrenics is associated with an immunological abnormality, but much work remains to be done before this is confirmed. A rigorously controlled situation is required to show that a substance obtained from the blood of schizophrenic patients can produce the symptoms of schizophrenia when injected into normal volunteers. We do not yet know the extent to which the abnormalities in blood found by physiochemical methods or by biological assays are specific to schizophrenia. Are they produced by chronic suffering and the conditions of institutionalization—such as repeated bouts of emotional distress, inadequate diet, and recurrent infections? This type of analytical problem regularly arises in research on severe mental disorders.

For about two decades, psychiatrists, psychologists, and sociologists have been interested in the families of schizophrenic patients. Much attention has been directed to the question of whether there are distinctive patterns of interaction that characterize such families. Several possibilities have been recognized: (1) Stressful family relationships might trigger a schizophrenic episode, perhaps by impinging on an inherited abnormality. (2) Special patterns of interaction might evolve over the years as family members try to cope with an abnormal child, much as they would cope with a brain-damaged child. (3) Special characteristics of one or both parents might inadvertently create a very difficult environment for a particular child, thus playing an important role in causing some cases of schizophrenia.

The third of these possibilities has elicited most interest, perhaps to the neglect of the first two. We wish now to convey the flavor of this research, examining the possibility that family experiences may contribute to the development of schizophrenia—at least in a subgroup of this common, severe disorder. These studies have relied mainly upon clinical observations of family members discussing shared problems, while one member is a hospitalized patient. Typically, the patient joins his parents and sometimes a sibling in these interviews. In some studies, many interviews occur over a period of months or even years. An effort is made to reconstruct the main trends of the patient's development, characteristic family relations over the years, and areas of stress and conflict. The more recent of these studies tend to record systematically certain principal categories of current interaction among the family members.

Some investigators have utilized data not only from clinical interviews but also from psychological tests. Analysis of detailed transcripts showed that parents of schizophrenics, when compared with control groups of parents of adolescents or young adults suffering from conditions other than schizophrenia (chronic physical illnesses and other psychiatric conditions), have certain specific defects in communication. Raters working "blind" on such transcripts were able to differentiate reliably (1) parents of young adult schizophrenics, (2) parents of childhood schizophrenics, and (3) parents of childhood neurotics.

Since communicative styles differ among various social groups, the defects found in such families have recently been examined in several types of low-income families. This was of special interest because the earlier studies were done largely with middle-class families. Family Rorschach test techniques were used with low-income families of white schizophrenics, low-income families of Negro schizophrenics, and low-income Negro control families (no schizophrenic member). Raters were able to differentiate the families of schizophrenics (of both races) from the Negro controls at a high level of statistical significance. Thus, the distinctive features of families with a schizophrenic member tend to occur in various socioeconomic classes and various ethnic groups.

Many investigators in the United States and Europe have studied interpersonal relationships in the families of schizophrenic patients and have compared them with normal families and families in which an adolescent or young adult has some chronic, nonschizophrenic psychiatric or medical problem. Each group of workers has noted distinctive features of relationships in the families of schizophrenics. Though each research group has evolved its own descriptive terms for these abnormalities, their basic findings are quite similar. One such finding is that the schizophrenic family member has, since childhood, had severely restricted opportunity for corrective experiences from the surrounding community. Parents of schizophrenics tend to block or undermine their efforts to reach out for new experiences, especially new relationships of a relatively intimate nature.

Apparently these parents are motivated in part by a wish to keep the patient intimately bound up with themselves. This may be particularly true of certain mothers who are lonely, alienated, and low in self-esteem. Such tendencies are accentuated by at least two characteristic problems of the parents' own relationship, reported by various investigators: (1) severe and enduring conflict between the parents; and (2) communication patterns that are not so clear and comprehensible as those observed between the parents of normal persons. To the extent that such difficulties are serious and persistent, they do not provide the offspring with a promising model for close human relationships. This effect is especially important for the child who has been selected for particularly intense involvement with the deeply troubled parent(s).

Some workers have compared psychotic and nonpsychotic offspring within a single family to see what aspects of family life either predispose toward or protect against illness. They report that offspring who later become schizophrenic often have a special meaning for their families and elicit an intense focusing of attention. Sometimes such a child is assigned a highly specialized role within the family, a role characterized by great demands on the child but allowing him little room for changing interests or values. He tends to be much more restricted in relations outside the family than do siblings who do not become schizophrenic. The latter tend to be more independent than the former, especially in relation to the mother.

Some families have been described in which the transmission of irrationality can be traced from parents to children. In such families, there is much evidence of bizarre thinking and paranoid attitudes. When such tendencies are linked with efforts to minimize a child's contacts with the world beyond the family, they pose a very difficult developmental situation.

In general, these family studies have meshed with a great deal of clinical observation in psychiatry, documenting the ways in which family environments shape the development of self-esteem, interpersonal relationships, and emotional response tendencies. Indeed, this special interest has become one of the most distinctive features of modern psychiatry. While the family environment has been shown beyond reasonable doubt to be of enormous importance in personality development, other environmental influences have been somewhat neglected. For example, peer relations outside the family—even in childhood and certainly in adolescence—must have a strong bearing on individual behavior. Recent social changes probably accentuate such influences—for example, the powerful "youth culture."

The family studies we have been describing—oriented toward causal factors in schizophrenia—are very difficult and methodologically complex. There is a growing awareness of the problems that need to be solved in order for these studies to have dependable, causal significance. These methodological problems deserve our attention, especially since they illustrate common problems in psychological and social research.

One problem is in selection of families for study. Ideally, families would be drawn at random from the entire pool of families containing a schizophrenic member. This would be difficult at best, and current practice is far from the ideal. It is quite possible that families are selected for these studies just because they give preliminary indications of interesting family dynamics. In any event, the early work in this field understandably offered little control of observer bias, either in selection of families or in recording of data.

If the patients have spent years in hospitals, the effects of such experience on the family may confound the issue. Since the studies are mainly cross-sectional and do not precede the illness, it is difficult to sort out family patterns that may have shaped the child's behavior in a schizophrenic direction from family patterns that arose in response to exceedingly difficult or bizarre behavior of the child. In any case, it is valuable for clinicians to know whether special patterns of interaction are likely to be found in families with a schizophrenic member, regardless of whether these patterns have causal significance.

In an effort to meet these methodological problems, current research shows the following trends:

1. Systematic observation and recording of data in specified categories.
2. "Blind" coding by multiple observers or raters, with statistical assessment of interobserver agreement.
3. Utilization of standardized measures to compare S families (those having a schizophrenic member) with non-S families—matched for age, sex, social class or ethnic group, and other relevant characteristics.
4. Systematic comparison of parents' relations to schizophrenic and nonschizophrenic offspring within a given family.
5. Matching of comparison groups on duration of hospitalization, with primary attention being given to those hospitalized only a short time prior to study.
6. Giving explicit attention to sampling considerations, in an effort to determine what proportion of S families can be expected to show each pattern.
7. Experimental analysis of interactions among family members to test, in a controlled situation, prevalent hypotheses about patterns of interaction in families with schizophrenic members. By bringing the mother, father, and schizophrenic offspring into the experimental research setting, the investigators seek to rigorously check the hypotheses regarding the schizophrenic family derived from clinical, descriptive studies.

Family studies in schizophrenia have already made several contributions. They have highlighted the potential value of studying the family as a unit, stimulating the development of a new form of treatment called conjoint psychotherapy, or family therapy. There has not yet been sufficient time to rigorously evaluate the effectiveness of such treatment. Family studies have drawn attention to subtle and complex patterns of communication and interpersonal relationships within the family. These observations and concepts may have value in the study of other kinds of groups—in therapeutic, educational, and work situations. In addition, they provide guidelines for prospective, longitudinal studies that may inform us not only about the genesis of schizophrenia but about much else in coping behavior and personality development. (See the later sections of this report, Disorders of Childhood, Development of Aggressive Behavior, Coping and Adaptation.) Though longitudinal studies are necessarily difficult, time-consuming, and expensive, they have great importance for the ultimate understanding of human behavior. It would be particularly desirable for psychiatry to take the initiative in mounting interdisciplinary, longitudinal studies of behavior development— linking medicine with behavioral sciences in the effort.

Much data indicates that psychiatric disorders of many types occur more often in the relatives of schizophrenics than in the relatives of neurotic patients or of normal persons. It is plausible that differences in severity of family psychopathology during the years of growth and development may account for some of these findings. However, much the same sort of evidence has been used to support the proposition that there is an inherited tendency toward schizophrenia. It is not possible from the studies described above to provide definitive clarification of genetic and environmental factors in the development of schizophrenia.

While these family environment studies have been evolving, genetic studies have been pursued on a parallel track. For many years, the main body of evidence cited in support of genetic influences in schizophrenia came from twin studies. However, these pioneering studies—much like the pioneering family environment studies—had serious methodological limitations, especially in lack of control for observer bias. In general, the twin studies and genetically oriented family studies pointed toward one major conclusion: the closer the biological relationship to an index case (diagnosed schizophrenic patient), the more likely is a person to suffer from schizophrenia (that is, the greater the concordance). There has recently been a "second wave" of twin and family studies, utilizing improved techniques of diagnosis, sampling, and determining concordance. In general, their results support the earlier work, but the concordance rates are lower. Thus, they suggest large roles for both heredity and environment. But they are not able to go far toward specifying the nature of gene-environment interactions.

Some workers have studied identical twins who are discordant for schizophrenia—that is, one twin suffers from the disorder, but the other twin does not. Here the genetic factors are presumably identical, and this provides an opportunity to identify distinctive environmental factors to which one twin has been exposed but the other has not. Both biological and interpersonal variables can be examined in this way, throwing new light on possible causal factors in schizophrenia. The method can also be useful in relation to other psychiatric problems.

Another approach to clarifying genetic and environmental factors has been the study of identical twins reared apart from very early in life—ideally from birth onward. Such cases are extremely interesting but very difficult to find; hence samples are small. The development of twin registries and television appeals have been helpful in locating twins reared apart.

Quite recently, an important set of studies has been conducted utilizing a new approach. These studies center on children adopted in infancy. Since these children are not reared by their biological parents, hereditary factors are separated from those of personal experience and family environment. In one study, two groups of carefully matched individuals reared in unrelated adoptive homes were compared: those who had a schizophrenic biological parent (index cases), and those who had nonschizophrenic biological parents. The prevalence of schizophrenia and related disorders among the index adoptees was considerably higher than among the control group (confirming the findings of an earlier study on foster-home–reared children). Interestingly, in these new studies the related disorders covered a considerable range of psychiatric manifestations. Thus, whatever is inherited is probably not schizophrenia per se, but some vulnerability that predisposes the child to a spectrum of disorders.

In a second study, the frequency and severity of psychopathology among parents who reared their own schizophrenic offspring was found to be significantly greater than among adoptive parents of a group of schizophrenic patients, which in turn was greater than among adoptive parents of nonschizophrenics. In the third study of this set, schizophrenia and related disorders were found to be randomly distributed in the adoptive families of a group of index cases (adoptees who became schizophrenic) and in the families of a control group (matched adoptees). However, the biological families of the index cases showed a significantly higher prevalence of schizophrenia and related disorders than the biological families of the controls.

Overall, the higher prevalence of psychopathology among the adoptees with an affected biological parent and among the biological parents and relatives of affected adoptees supports the concept of an important inherited component in the disorder. These studies provide the most clear-cut evidence so far available of genetic factors predisposing to the development of schizophrenia.

It is no longer worth while to ask, Is schizophrenia genetic or environmental in origin? The basic questions now center on the specific nature of gene-environment interactions. Can the inherited tendency be detected by some peculiarity of behavior in childhood? By what biochemical mechanisms do the genes affect the brain and hence behavior? What experiences in the family or in other environmental situations are likely to elicit full expression of the genetic tendency? And what experiences are likely to counteract it, thus diminishing the risk of psychosis? In search of answers to such questions, it will be necessary to mount prospective, longitudinal studies in which genetic, biochemical, neurophysiological, personality, family, and community variables can be studied over a period of years, dating from early life of the subjects. Many investigators favor a general working hypothesis that integrates biological and psychosocial factors. For example, it may be that adverse interpersonal experience triggers the onset of overt schizophrenic behavior in persons made susceptible by a genetically determined biochemical abnormality in neuroregulatory processes.

A decade ago, a survey of the persons treated for mental illness in one American community had a great impact on the entire mental health field. It has become a classic analysis of social environment and mental illness, and has stimulated much further research. The distribution of schizophrenic patients among the various social classes was a crucial part of the study, as were the differing ways in which these patients were treated, depending on their social class. This was a collaborative study conducted by sociologists and psychiatrists in search of answers to two important questions: Is mental illness related to social class? Do patients from different social classes receive different kinds of treatment?

This research group undertook to study all the psychiatric patients in treatment in their community at a particular time, the institutions where they were being treated, and the individuals treating them. While members of all social classes in the community were found in all categories of mental illness, the predominant type of illness dif-

fered according to s
more prevalent in the
schizophrenic patients fro
attitudes toward mental ill
families of upper-class patients
ministered and the patient's resp
related to his socioeconomic status
were much more frequently given psy
the lower classes were more frequently tr
as electroconvulsive therapy. (See also th
The rate of recovery and return to the co
the upper classes. Among other findings, this re
the class-linked nature of psychiatric services and p
toward more equitable distribution of mental health
drew attention to the potential value of epidemiologic
clarifying psychiatric problems.

Most of the studies sketched in this section deal dir
schizophrenic patients. However, it seems likely that the t
clarification of such a complex disorder will depend on a broad
of scientific understanding. Investigators concerned with sch
phrenia must scan persistently for the relevance of newly emerging
basic information on brain, behavior, and social environment. Most
students of the problem believe that complex interactions of biological and psychosocial processes will prove to be crucial in schizophrenia. The relevant basic sciences include fields so diverse as genetics,
biochemistry, neurophysiology, endocrinology, anthropology, psychology, sociology, and epidemiology. (For additional research on
schizophrenia, see the section, Sleep and Dreaming.)

DEPRESSION

Depressions are common disorders. In community sur-
veys, prevalence rates for depression have been found to be slightly
under 1 per 1000 population for depressive psychoses, and two to
three times that for depressive neuroses. This means that, as a rough
estimate, about half a million Americans are suffering from clinical
depression at any given time (that is, distress more severe than the
transient sadness of everyday life). More than 300,000 people were
treated for depression during the past year in the United States.

19,000
most of
icide is
which
equent

ch the
essions
l cate-
ic de-

. It is
lpless-
. The
such
andly
rying
him.
also
both

less
less-
low-

... often the patient

... to perform his job or carry out household tasks, albeit with difficulty.

Masked depression is a condition in which the basic, underlying mood disorder is obscured by prominent bodily complaints such as insomnia, constipation, loss of appetite, and headaches. Though these masked depressions are quite common in medical practice, they have been the subject of surprisingly little systematic research.

The problems of depression and suicide are closely linked, yet suicide is only one of the serious manifestations of the depressive illnesses. Clinical experience suggests that depression predisposes to alcoholism and to serious accidents. Many physicians feel that depression increases susceptibility to a wide range of disease processes. Altogether, the depressions may well be one of the most important and neglected public health problems of our time.

In recent years there has been a gradual accumulation of evidence suggesting a link between depression and brain biogenic amine metabolism. While this linkage has not been definitively established, it has provoked much careful research and drawn scientific interest to these significant problems. Much interest has centered on the catecholamines. The catecholamines of importance in mammalian brains are noradrenalin and a related compound, dopamine. Quite recently, adrenalin, too, has taken on a significance in brain function. A decade's research has shown that the catecholamines are involved in the transmission of information from one nerve cell to another in many regions of the brain, especially those that mediate emotional behavior. Several important drugs bring about their clinical effects by affecting the action of the catecholamines in the brain.

Much neurophysiological, neuroanatomical and behavioral evidence has identified specific regions of the brain that are crucial in mediating emotional experience. These areas include the hypothalamus, near the base of the brain, and the limbic system. These regions are much older in evolution than the cerebral cortex that surrounds them. With the development of chemical methods for the estimation of catecholamine tissue concentrations, it has become clear that noradrenalin is localized in the brain areas concerned with emotional behavior.

Meanwhile, reserpine (the first major tranquilizer) came into clinical use in the treatment of hypertension (high blood pressure). Two interesting facts about this drug gradually emerged: it often induced depression as a side effect, and it depleted animal brains of catecholamines. This raised the question of whether low amine levels at certain sites in the brain might be associated with depression. A great many laboratory and clinical studies followed this line. Drugs that caused depletion and inactivation of brain noradrenalin sometimes cause behavioral sedation or depression; on the other hand, drugs that increase or potentiate brain noradrenalin tend, under proper testing conditions, to be associated with behavioral stimulation or excitement. The latter drugs often have an antidepressant effect in man. Hence, a catecholamine hypothesis of affective (mood) disorders has arisen: some depressions may be associated with a relative deficiency of noradrenalin at functionally important receptor sites in the brain, whereas some excited states may be associated with an excess of such amines. This hypothesis is consistent with much of the available evidence, and is currently provoking careful research; but it has not yet been rigorously established, and is presented here as an illustration of an important hypothesis undergoing study. This caution is necessary since there are other explanations of the same data which invoke other mechanisms, such as turnover of the amines, and would lead to different conclusions.

Confirmation of any biochemical hypothesis ultimately requires specific demonstration of the biochemical abnormality in the naturally occurring human disorder. Workers in this field have been confronted with a great barrier: how to determine biochemical events in the human brain from measurements of available body fluids, mainly urine and blood. Several years of basic research in laboratory animals showed that one compound, methoxyhydroxyphenylglycol (MHPG), offers promise. A definite fraction of MHPG in urine is derived from brain noradrenalin. (So far this has not been true of any other amine metabolite; the others reflect events in peripheral tissues rather than brain.) The applicability of this basic finding to man was studied next. The catecholamine hypothesis predicts that severely depressed patients excrete less MHPG in their urine than do nondepressed persons, if MHPG does indeed reflect brain amine metabolism. So, catecholamine derivatives were measured in the urine of severely depressed patients and normal individuals, and it was found that the group of depressed patients had significantly lower levels of MHPG in urine than did the control subjects, while the two groups did not differ in other urinary catecholamine derivatives. These results will no doubt serve to spur further investigation along this line.

Of great importance is the finding that lithium carbonate is effective in the treatment of manic states (see the section, Pharmacotherapy) and in some depressive states as well. The mechanism by which this chemical compound acts is still unresolved; links to the neuroregulatory agents are currently being investigated. Here, as elsewhere, a distinctive behavioral effect produced by a drug may provide a lead toward investigation of underlying biochemical processes and hence to the fundamental nature of the disorder.

Some investigators have challenged the catecholamine hypothesis, pointing out that much of the evidence is indirect and could implicate other neuroregulatory agents as well. For example, changes have been reported in the level of serotonin in the brain. (Serotonin is a member of another significant class of brain amines, the indoleamines; see the sections, Schizophrenia and Sleep and Dreaming.) The demonstration of a biochemical abnormality in brain amines might well imply a genetically determined enzymatic defect in a stress-responsive system. Some clinical investigations have indicated an inherited tendency toward depressive responses. Other possibilities also require investigation. Some animal research indicates that early experiences of the immature organism may cause enduring biochemical changes. Such environmentally induced changes might predispose some individuals to depression in later years. In any event, it is unlikely that the metabolism of brain amines will tell the whole story of the depressions. These amines at crucial sites in the brain may well be of great importance in the regulation of emotional experience. But many other biochemical, physiological, and psychological factors will have to be examined experimentally and clinically before a comprehensive account of the depressions can be documented. Further, the relationship between these various factors will have to be examined. A major area in which information will have to be obtained is the way in which psychological factors and biochemical factors interact. How do psychological states influence brain chemistry and how does that change in brain chemistry influence further behavior? There may be a cyclical relationship with many feedback controls that relate biochemical events and psychological events. This area has been largely unexplored.

One interesting line of clinical investigation has centered on the circumstances that precipitate or exacerbate depressive episodes. These studies have dealt with relations of personal loss, grief, and clinical depression. Patients very often come to psychiatric attention in the context of an important loss—of a person with whom a highly significant relationship had existed, or of an important source of self-esteem (such as, a valued position). The most vivid instance is the grief reaction to the loss of a personally significant individual.

The appearance of persons in acute grief is vivid. The main features are sensations of bodily distress occurring in waves lasting from twenty minutes to an hour at a time, a feeling of tightness in the throat, a choking sensation with shortness of breath, deep sighing, a sensation of emptiness, a feeling of profound weakness, and an intense subjective distress involving a feeling of agonizing, irretrievable loss.

Thus, grief presents a specific pattern of distress precipitated by a personally significant loss. The person's focus is on this loss. Usually, there is gradual recovery through a difficult process of mourning. This recovery occurs over a period of some weeks to months. However, some persons go on to a clinical depression, in which there is a pervasive undermining of interests, activities, and interpersonal relations, with feelings of despondency.

There is a problem of differential susceptibility to grief. For many years, clinicians have had the impression that grief is one of the major precipitating factors in neurotic and psychotic depressive reactions. Many psychiatrists believe that loss of a valued person—loss not only through death but also through separation, divorce, and for other reasons—is the principal class of precipitating circumstances in the psychiatric depressions. Yet most people experience such losses at one time or another and feel considerable emotional distress. What factors make some people break down and become incapacitated by depression? We simply do not yet know with scientific adequacy, but brain biochemistry might well have a significant bearing on vulnerability to loss.

A related set of factors currently under growing investigation are neuroendocrine relations (the relationships between the brain and hormones secreted by the internal glands of the body). The older concept of psychiatric depression as characterized by a general slowing of activity throughout a wide variety of physiologic systems is giving way to data showing substantial elevations in hormones of great biological potency. Elevated levels of the principal hormone of the adrenal cortex are often observed in clinical depression. Elevations in thyroid hormone also tend to occur when depression is severe, but are less striking than the changes in adrenal steroids. Such elevations in adrenal hormone levels may be sustained or recurrent for weeks, or even months, if the depression persists. The extent of hormone elevation is closely related to the degree of distress and, in turn, to the effectiveness of coping behavior. Adrenocortical steroids and their metabolites have been shown (mainly in animal studies but to some extent in man as well) to be capable of affecting brain function and behavior. Variations in metabolism of these hormones may have a bearing on the individual's response to major disappointments and personal losses.

Recent studies have described the impressive variety and usual effectiveness of patterns of coping behavior through which problems of personal loss are normally met. (See the section, Coping and Adaptation.) These studies further accentuate the question of differential susceptibility to loss and grief. What goes wrong behaviorally and physiologically in those who become overwhelmed with despondency? This should be a major line of psychiatric research in the next decade.

It is likely that differentiation within the broad group of depressions will become increasingly possible on various grounds: behavioral, genetic, pharmacological, biochemical, and neurophysiological. On whatever basis, such differentiation is likely to enhance our understanding and increase our effectiveness in dealing with these common and serious disorders. The same may well be true of the schizophrenias. As has proven to be the case in mental retardation, there may be a number of different pathways through which a common clinical result can be achieved. (For additional research on depression, see the section, Sleep and Dreaming.)

DISORDERS IN CHILDHOOD

Child development research has become an exciting discipline, cutting across biological, psychological, and social approaches, and including psychiatry. In the future, this may well be one of the most important areas in the study of behavior, particularly because it has so much potential for the prevention of human suffering. As scientific knowledge of development and deviations increases, the effectiveness of preventive approaches will be greatly augmented. We can only give a brief illustration here of promising areas.

Evidence has accumulated showing that poor maternal health during pregnancy increases hazards to the unborn child. Complications of pregnancy are much more common among poor people than among others. These complications are associated with insufficient medical care, inadequate nutrition, unsatisfactory living conditions, and psychological stress. In these circumstances there is an increased risk of reproductive casualties such as stillbirth, cerebral palsy, convulsive disorders, mental retardation, and behavior disorders. Premature birth is also commoner among mothers living in poverty, and is accompanied by increased risk of later behavior pathology.

Important research on attachment behavior has been conducted by students of both child development and animal behavior. These studies have shown how enduring attachments are formed in early life, and have revealed the very unfortunate consequences of disruption of such attachments. One line of inquiry has dealt with the consequences of inadequate maternal behavior for the child's physical and behavioral development. Repeatedly, psychiatrists, psychologists, and pediatricians have documented a syndrome of intellectual retardation and emotional disturbance that follows upon incompetent mothering. The most extreme form of deprivation of mothering leads to failure to gain weight, retarded development, even sometimes to emaciation and death. With good hospital care, even emaciated children tend to recover rapidly unless the condition prior to hospitalization has been very prolonged. Maternal deprivation that is less severe but yet persistent has been linked to deficient performance on intelligence tests in later life and to difficulties in forming close relations with other persons throughout life. We need no longer assume that early separation of mother and infant, or even loss of the mother, in and of itself, necessarily leads to permanent damage. Much depends on the adequacy of substitute mothering. Recent research has attempted to sort out the various factors that have an influence on long-term outcome when early separation or loss occurs. Workers in this field have had stimulating interactions with those conducting the monkey experiments on maternal deprivation referred to elsewhere in this report.

Unfortunately, many children are exposed to risks of neglect and deprivation. More than two million children in the United States live in very poor socioeconomic conditions in which the family environment is marginal. A large proportion of very poor families are in fact multiple problem families, suffering from chronic handicaps—physical, psychiatric, and social. Moreover, about a quarter of a million children are in foster homes, designed to provide adequate family care for orphaned or abandoned children. But studies in this area have highlighted the inadequacy of many (though by no means all) such placements. Therefore, some current experimentation seeks to define living arrangements that might provide the necessary human attachments and stimulation for children without parents. These institutions would be much smaller and more individualized than traditional orphanages.

Clinical observations have long suggested that strongly unwanted children are especially likely to become emotionally disturbed. Birth control and family planning programs could reduce the occurrence of such high risk children. Yet the advent of improved birth control technology has not led to such rapid progress as had been generally expected. Since the population problem is so crucial in modern society, there is an urgent need for psychological and social research on adult attitudes, values, and fears that impede effective use of family planning methods.

During the past few years, pediatricians and child psychiatrists have been surprised by the frequent appearance of the "battered child." They see children who are badly beaten, often to the point of multiple fractures, by enraged parents. Indeed, the injuries are sometimes fatal. Clinical investigations are attempting to identify the distinctive characteristics of such parents, the conditions under which severe beatings are likely to occur, and ways to prevent the carnage. It is notable that child abuse is not linked to social class, ethnic or religious variables.

Much careful research has been done on a particular neurotic disorder of childhood, school phobia. This reaction appears to be a special case of separation anxiety. It can be treated effectively in children of elementary school age with lasting results found in follow-up study. The same syndrome has been much more difficult to treat in adolescence, and tends to become chronic if untreated. Therapeutic effectiveness is linked to promptness of intervention. Yet, there is typically much delay before such patients reach a clinic, and often more delay (because of clinic waiting lists) before treatment begins. This points up the need for studies on screening methods that could provide early warning signals among school children. Here, as elsewhere, the most promising approach combines early detection with prompt intervention. We anticipate an upsurge of prevention-oriented research in the school years. One direction of such research, so far seriously neglected in psychiatry, is the early detection of persons prone to violence. (This is discussed in the later section, Development of Aggressive Behavior.)

The most severe disorders with which child psychiatrists deal are the childhood psychoses or childhood schizophrenias. Fortunately, such illnesses occur but rarely. The family with a psychotic child is sorely burdened, and at present psychiatry can hold out little hope for improvement in the child's condition. The most severe form, early infantile autism, has its onset in the earliest years of life. Other forms emerge during the third and later years, although often the illness is not diagnosed until the child enters school, where his abnormal and bizarre behavior quickly arouses concern. The child's relations with other persons, including members of his family, are markedly atypical, usually distant and impersonal. He may be mute; if he does talk, his speech is unusual. His day-to-day behavior may center on a few acts, performed repetitively. Changes in his environment or routines may set off extreme outbursts of anger. Current research on these children—including careful observational studies, attempts at drug therapy, and the use of conditioning techniques to aid their unlearning of maladaptive behavior and their learning of new skills—may yield information that will aid in their treatment and shed new light on normal human development.

Concern with the socioeconomically disadvantaged child has spurred vigorous efforts along several important lines of research. First, research into the intellectual development of children has been greatly intensified and a special effort has been made to discover the optimal learning environment for the young child. Head Start programs for disadvantaged children are being set up and evaluated for their effectiveness in preparing children for school. Second, concepts derived from research on the impact of observer bias on the outcome of laboratory experiments have been employed in social psychological studies in the classroom. Experiments have shown that a teacher's expectation and bias markedly influence the student's achievement—low expectation yields low performance. The implications of this for the education of disadvantaged children are now being clarified. Finally, there is great interest in studying the distinctive cognitive styles of disadvantaged children in an effort to understand the nature of their learning disability. This work aims to reverse the present trend in which these children show progressive decrements in achievement as they proceed through the school years. Such research involves a conjunction of psychiatric and educational work; some encouraging collaborations have recently emerged.

3
RESEARCH ON PSYCHIATRIC TREATMENT

Psychiatrists employ diverse strategies to treat their patients. Two are especially prominent and have served as the focus of considerable investigation: pharmacotherapy and psychotherapy. In this chapter, we consider what research has revealed about their uses and effectiveness.

PHARMACOTHERAPY

One of the central responsibilities of psychiatric research—as in other clinical fields—is to provide dependable assessments of the efficacy and safety of the various therapeutic measures undertaken in the discipline. For psychiatry, such assessment refers mainly to drug treatment and psychotherapy. Some similar issues are involved in the two areas, but the task is less complex in drug treatment. So we shall begin by describing briefly a well-designed study of the effects of drugs on mental disorder. This study is an example of recent research in the field which has relied heavily on the collaboration of psychiatrists and psychologists.

Several drugs of the phenothiazine group have been developed in the past decade and have been utilized in treating schizophrenic disorders. They are often referred to as major tranquilizers. The best known is chlorpromazine. Early clinical experience with these drugs was generally encouraging. A difference of opinion arose among clinical observers as to whether each drug was specifically effective with a particular subgroup of schizophrenic patients. A research group then undertook a large-scale experiment to put this possibility to a rigorous test. They enlisted the collaboration of various hospitals across the country. This collaboration permitted pooling of information on an adequate scale and tended to eliminate the influence of unusual circumstances at a particular hospital. A crucial concept in this experiment was that it followed a double-blind design. The patients were assigned at random to treatment with one of the drugs or to a placebo. The various capsules were coded so that neither the patient, the physicians, nor the nurses knew which drug (or placebo) was being used until the study was finished six weeks later. All patients received typical supportive assistance in the hospital, regardless of the treatment to which they were assigned. When the code was broken at the end of the study, it was noted that the patients who improved on one of the drugs had had a different pattern of pretreatment symptoms than did the patients who improved on any other drug. In short, the improvers on each drug could be identified by a unique pattern of pretreatment symptoms. For example, acetophenazine was most effective for paranoid-excited patients and chlorpromazine was most effective in patients with incoherent speech. The findings are already clinically useful, and they highlight the potential utility for future research of differentiating within common diagnostic categories.

Double-blind methodology has been extremely valuable in achieving objectivity in drug research. If an investigator knows what drug his patient is getting, there is considerable risk that he may inadvertently produce a "placebo effect"—an improvement in the patient's condition caused not by the drug itself but by circumstances surrounding its administration. Important factors that may contribute to a "placebo effect" are the patient's wish for improvement, spontaneous remission of the disorder, the medical staff's enthusiasm for the drug, additional attention and care given the patient along with the drug, and inadvertent observer bias favoring drug efficacy. For reasons of this sort, research on drug effects has benefited greatly from an experimental design in which neither the patient nor the therapeutic staff knows which medication has been given until the study period is over and all behavioral observations have been recorded. Some investigators have reviewed the research literature on psychopharmacology and found that uncontrolled studies consistently give a more encouraging evaluation of drug effect than controlled studies. Uncontrolled studies often give enthusiastic reports about drugs later proven to be useless; less often, uncontrolled observations suggest that a drug is useless, only to have controlled studies later show it to be valuable. Thus, methodological problems in drug research deserve much attention in future work. For the summary of current knowledge on clinically significant drug effects in schizophrenia and depression, we rely entirely on controlled studies utilizing double-blind design.

The following questions have come under scrutiny in psychopharmacology. Is a particular drug better than a placebo in treating a certain disorder? If several drugs are promising in the treatment of this disorder, is one better than the others? If drugs of roughly equal effectiveness are available, does one have fewer undesirable side effects? Do subgroups of a particular disorder respond differently to different drugs? What dosage and duration are optimal for a given condition, considering both short-term recovery and long-term recurrence? When single drugs fail, will a combination work? What effects may be produced by the social context in which a drug is administered? What are the circumstances in which drug treatment may facilitate psychotherapy?

Studies of hospitalized schizophrenic patients clearly indicate that the major tranquilizers, particularly those of the phenothiazine group, have made a substantial contribution to therapeutic effectiveness. Very likely, this has been a significant factor in the decline of mental hospital populations in recent years—the first time this has happened in American history. Within the phenothiazine group, a number of drugs are about equally effective in treatment of the broad group of schizophrenics: chlorpromazine, perphenazine, triflupromazine, fluphenazine, trifluoperazine, prochlorperazine, and thioridazine. They are somewhat more effective than mepazine and promazine. All of these phenothiazines are more effective than placebo or phenobarbital. It should be noted that the early successes of the major tranquilizers helped to transform the social environment of mental hospitals. Patients were viewed more optimistically and with less fear. This in turn improved the interpersonal climate and encouraged other therapeutic approaches.

Patients started on tranquilizers in the hospital have been followed up after leaving the hospital, sometimes for long periods, in order to determine the therapeutic regimen that offers greatest protection against serious relapse. These studies consistently show that when a phenothiazine is discontinued within a few months after discharge, there is a considerably greater risk of relapse. This relapse tendency is much more striking in some patients than in others. An important line of future inquiry will be the effort to identify the most vulnerable patients. Some aspects of personality and current social environment are clearly relevant; perhaps drug metabolism is also. Studies of schizophrenic patients treated on an outpatient basis show phenothiazines to be more effective than placebo in reducing psychotic symptoms and reducing the need for hospitalization.

Gradually, distinctions within the group of phenothiazines have been emerging: (1) Certain drugs tend to be most effective with a particular subgroup of schizophrenic patients. (2) The frequency and nature of undesirable side effects differs a good deal from one phenothiazine drug to another. (3) The chemical processing (metabolism) of a given drug in the body differs a good deal from one person to another. These differences are derived to some extent from inherited differences in the enzymes in the body that are important in disposing of drugs. Thus, the new science of pharmacogenetics deserves serious consideration in relation to psychiatric problems. In other areas of medicine, pharmacogenetics has given insights into the biochemical basis for certain disorders. Advances of this sort have taken place when clinicians and biochemists worked together, first sorting out a clinical subgroup on the basis of an aberrant drug response, and then going on to characterize the biochemical abnormality underlying the response. A similar course may well be followed in the next decade of psychiatric research.

After encouraging results of drug therapy in schizophrenia became apparent, there was a renewal of interest in finding drugs to treat depression. Here, too, an initial phase of hopeful assertions based on uncontrolled studies was followed by a sobering period in which serious questions arose about both safety and efficacy of the drugs—particularly a group of compounds known as monoamine oxidase inhibitors.

More recently, another group of drugs, the tricyclic compounds, has come out well in double-blind studies. In this latter group, there is now consistent evidence for the effectiveness of imipramine, amitriptyline, and phenelzine in the treatment of patients who are hospitalized because of moderately severe depressions. The rare studies which failed to find a beneficial effect were usually done either with insufficient dosage or with a very small sample of patients.

Despite high rates of improvement associated with these drugs, followup studies have shown high relapse rates. In one study of patients successfully treated with antidepressant medication and maintained on medication for at least six months after discharge, 25 percent were readmitted to the hospital at least once within eighteen months. The problem of suicide during treatment is still a serious one. So, significant progress has been made in drug therapy of depression, but much remains to be done.

Some studies have compared these drugs with electroconvulsive therapy (ECT, or electroshock therapy), which has long been known to be effective in very severe depressions. One careful, systematic study showed that ECT produced more improvement in severely depressed, highly suicidal patients than did imipramine, phenelzine, isocarboxazid, or placebo. However, there are as yet only a few adequately controlled studies making systematic comparisons of various antidepressant therapies in different groups of depressed patients. Such studies are badly needed.

In the acutely suicidal, depressed patient, ECT is especially useful because of its rapidity of action. In recent years, its unpleasant side effects have been diminished by the use of short-acting anaesthetics and muscle relaxants; both the discomfort to the patient and the dangers of the technique have been reduced. However, significant disadvantages remain. Compared with drugs, the treatment is expensive; it requires considerable time of highly trained personnel. Most patients find the procedure quite unpleasant although it is not painful. There is loss of memory which is initially quite extensive; some amnesia may persist for long periods. It is best restricted to hospital use. Intensive efforts are currently under way to find chemical agents at least as useful as ECT without its undesirable concomitant features.

Quite recently, lithium salts have been shown to be remarkably effective in reducing severe excitement and agitation. These effects have been impressive in the manic conditions heretofore quite resistant to therapy. Their value in the treatment of depression in manic-depressive patients is still undetermined. Long-term followup studies are needed, especially in regard to possible prevention of manic recurrences. Very recently, preliminary evidence has emerged suggesting the value of lithium in preventing recurrence of both manic and depressive phases of manic-depressive psychoses.

With respect to drugs used in psychiatric treatment, just as with

drugs used in other medical treatments, we need a better understanding of the basic mechanisms by which the drugs work in the
body. In drug research in all branches of medicine, once the mechanism of action is well understood, improved forms of the drug can
be developed. The needed basic research includes investigations of
the behavioral effects in animals of a diversity of drugs and of their
mechanisms of action. We need also to investigate the physiological
effects of the drugs and their effects on specific biochemical processes
in the brain. Further, we need studies in which variations in the
chemical structure of a drug are related to variations in its action.
The need for studies of this sort points up the need for more
knowledge of the fundamental problems of several sciences.

The time lag between the basic discovery of drugs that hold
promise for psychiatry and their clinical application is often surprisingly short. For many drugs it has been considerably less than a
decade. Altogether, the quality of research in psychopharmacology
has rapidly improved during the past decade, and its clinical yield
is certainly encouraging. But this is a new area for science, and
much of its promise remains to be fulfilled.

PSYCHOTHERAPY

Research on psychotherapy is similar in principle to research on pharmacotherapy, but in practice the difficulties of the
former have been much greater. One of the main reasons for this
difficulty is that it has so far been possible to achieve only a pale
shadow of double-blind conditions. Because of inherent methodological limits, and a short scientific tradition in this area, there has
been ample room for observer bias and for placebo effects. Under
these circumstances, authority tends to substitute for evidence.
Claims and counter-claims, attacks and counter-attacks flourish when
it is very difficult to get decisive results through systematic controlled research.

Since the number of patients in psychotherapy with any one
psychiatrist tends to be modest, particularly in intensive psychotherapy, it is necessary to pool information in order to get sample
sizes large enough to permit meaningful statistical analysis. This
problem is even more acute in assessment of psychotherapy than in
psychopharmacology, where multiple-hospital collaborative studies

were possible. There has been some effort in the past decade to conduct systematic surveys of professional experience on a regional or even national basis in order to begin to cope with this problem. For example, a national survey of psychoanalytic experience was recently published in which it was possible to get some information on several thousand patients treated by eight hundred psychoanalysts. The data reported a fairly comprehensive picture of the socioeconomic status of patients in psychoanalytic treatment. The study also provided some information on the extent to which improvement was attained in various patient categories. However, the improvement estimates were based entirely on the judgment of the analyst conducting the treatment. While this is a useful first approximation, it is a long way from double-blind conditions. Still, it establishes a precedent for large-scale pooling of information on psychoanalytic treatment and provides a methodological analysis that could contribute to future improvements in such studies.

Another group of investigators utilized pooling of information from a sizeable number of patients and their psychotherapists in order to get a detailed retrospective view from each, particularly with regard to improvement. They found, as many other studies have found, a set of differences between socioeconomic classes in respect to psychotherapy. Patients from the lower socioeconomic classes are less likely than those from higher socioeconomic classes to be assigned to intensive psychotherapy oriented toward detailed understanding of personal problems. Patients from the lower classes are also more likely to have difficulty in communicating with professional psychotherapists. One important direction of effort during the next decade will probably be the search for conditions favoring effective communication across class and ethnic barriers. The results of this study, like many others, suggested that patients tend to benefit not only from an enhanced understanding of themselves, but also from certain qualities of the therapist, such as a genuine interest in and respect for the patient. The patients in this study, as in several others, were less concerned with the alleviation of specific symptoms than with an enhancement of a sense of competence and worth, and with improvements in their relations with other people.

Much controversy has occurred over the efficacy of psychotherapy, both in individual and group forms. There has been a tendency for enthusiastic assertions of great therapeutic benefit; and there have also been sweeping denunciations of psychotherapy. Unfortunately, the evidence from careful, systematic and even partially controlled studies is so limited that little can yet be said on firm scientific ground about effectiveness of psychotherapy. Certainly, clinical experience, though uncontrolled, has now accumulated on a large scale over the past two decades and is reasonably encouraging. Moreover, increasingly well-designed studies of therapeutic outcome have been appearing during the past few years, and they tend to give more favorable evidence than was previously available.

Some early critiques of psychotherapeutic effectiveness, based on the scanty research of a decade and more ago, drew very harsh conclusions and have been widely publicized. While these harsh critiques have been useful in challenging complacent assumptions and stimulating better research, it now seems likely that they were considerably overdrawn or at least premature in their conclusions. They were largely based on studies that had serious limitations because of the lack of control groups, the very brief treatment period, the fact that therapists were often inexperienced, and the unknown reliability and validity of measurement techniques. In the past few years, several well-designed studies have appeared, using various types of control groups, including placebo conditions. These studies at least convey a sense of movement in the direction of methodological refinement that should permit more adequate answers over the next decade.

One line of inquiry that can be anticipated is the effort to specify patient characteristics that are important in relation to a particular method of therapy. Clearly, the older studies that lumped together all kinds of patients, all kinds of therapists, and all modes of therapy have not been very informative, nor is there any reason to expect them to be so. Clinical experience, now partially supported by research evidence, suggests that a given type of therapy is likely to be beneficial for certain patients, has no effect on certain other patients, and has an appreciable risk of harmful effects on still other patients. Thus, here as elsewhere in psychiatric research, it is becoming increasingly important to sort out subgroups within broad clinical entities, if meaningful findings are to be established.

It is sometimes said that spontaneous recovery (recovery without professional intervention) occurs in about two-thirds of all categories. While this may be an attractive assumption, the scientific basis for it is certainly not apparent at present. On the contrary, it seems more likely that the spontaneous recovery rate varies remarkably across patient types. In most situations, it is by no means clear what baseline of spontaneous recovery should be utilized in order to obtain a meaningful comparison with therapeutic efforts. It remains largely for future research to determine differential spontaneous recovery rates and differential effects of treatment in various clinical conditions. In any event, there is general agreement that adequate assessment of effectiveness will rest upon consideration of multiple aspects of change in treatment. A person may change markedly in one respect while remaining unchanged in another. It will be necessary to specify various dimensions of change and to measure reliably the extent of change along each of these dimensions.

Recent research on individual psychotherapy points toward the following tentative conclusions: (1) Individuals in psychotherapy tend to become better or worse than similar individuals who do not receive treatment. Some individuals in control groups who receive no formal psychotherapy nevertheless derive benefit from informal therapeutic contacts with nonprofessional people who are highly significant to them. These facts make it very difficult to set up a no-therapy control group. It places a stringent but perhaps desirable challenge upon any formal therapeutic methods: they must produce results significantly better than the informal-therapy control group. (2) Improvement in therapy is not only a function of technique but also, importantly, of personal characteristics of the therapist, such as his interest, respect, and ability to understand what the patient is trying to convey. The extent of his professional experience also seems important. (3) Patients from relatively higher socioeconomic classes tend to benefit more than patients from lower socioeconomic classes. This seems due in large part to differences in values and expectations between lower-class patients and middle-class therapists. (4) Therapeutic effectiveness probably increases with clarity of the patient's expectations about the nature of the task in psychotherapy, including his relationship with the therapist.

Changes in the atmosphere of research on psychotherapy have plainly occurred. Narrow, doctrinaire preoccupations are no longer readily accepted, regardless of theoretical preference. The demand for data to back up therapeutic claims has increased notably. There is also a trend toward placing psychotherapeutic process in the broader context of behavioral science research. In this perspective, psychotherapy becomes one kind of social relationship, similar to others. Thus, bodies of information on human learning, social influence, and small-group interaction are pertinent to psychotherapy. There is a search for ways of conducting psychotherapy that will be more incisive and economical. One such approach that appears promising is based on prompt intervention in time of personal crisis. Similarly, there has been a sharp increase in clinical explorations of therapeutic groups; quite recently there has been an encouraging rise of systematic research on group therapy. These newer trends, arising mainly in a clinical context, pose a great challenge and opportunity for scientific investigation of individual and group psychotherapy in the next decade.

4
FUNDAMENTAL TOPICS IN PSYCHIATRIC RESEARCH

ANIMAL EXPERIMENTAL MODELS OF BEHAVIOR DISORDERS

The importance of early experience in shaping later behavior was given much emphasis by Freud and has been an important issue in clinical work. In recent years, a new experimental approach of great interest has come upon the scene. Experiments with monkeys and apes have provided important evidence that abnormal early rearing conditions can produce severe behavior disorders in adult life. Some of these disorders bear considerable resemblance to certain features of human psychotic behavior (as described in the earlier section on schizophrenia). In any event, they are intrinsically interesting and point out a promising pathway for psychiatric research of the future.

Let us therefore turn our attention briefly to the studies of nonhuman primates that have been quite important during the past decade and are likely to become even more so. These studies are significant in the behavioral sciences for two reasons: they provide our best insights into the evolution of human behavior, and they provide us with useful experimental models of behavior disorders. The pursuit of such research has now been greatly facilitated by a wise act of public policy—the establishment of seven regional primate research centers in the United States. A great impetus to our understanding of monkeys and apes has come from a few pioneering psychologists, zoologists, anthropologists, and psychiatrists who have studied nonhuman primates in their natural habitats as well as in laboratories.

In the field studies of nonhuman primates under natural condi-

57

tions, one of the most striking and consistent observations has been the extraordinary richness and diversity of interanimal contact during the years of growth and development. Recent laboratory investigations with caged primates have provided a stark and informative contrast. The most dramatic comparison is provided by social isolation experiments. The behavioral effects of raising rhesus macaque monkeys until early adolescence in total social isolation—including isolation from contact both with other monkeys and with man— have proven quite devastating. The effects include gross disruption of interanimal contact, especially withdrawal and avoidance of contact; crouching for very long periods with very few responses directed toward the environment; a variety of maladaptive, self-oriented behavior patterns, including persistent thumb-sucking, self-clasping and stereotyped rocking; self-punitive behavior, such as self-biting, particularly upon the approach of other animals. The effects of partial social isolation are similar, though less profound and somewhat reversible. Current research in this area includes an attempt to determine the minimal length of time of rearing in social isolation that will produce these profound effects, and a search for conditions under which such disturbance may be reversible. This area is ripe for the study of biological factors. Are there, for example, permanent effects on endocrine function?

Similar studies have been done on the effects of rearing chimpanzees in isolation for three years (during the infancy period). Peculiar stereotyped behavior patterns are produced by such deprivation. These patterns are already present in the deprivation chamber, before the animal is brought into contact with others. They are, however, markedly accentuated by novel and stressful experiences after he emerges. When the isolation-reared animal is placed with another chimpanzee of similar age, he avoids contact. He also shows emotional disturbances that interfere with his response on tests of learning ability. In general, isolation-reared infant chimpanzees differ enormously from infant chimpanzees reared by their mothers— especially those reared in their natural habitat.

These experimental animals, studied six to nine years after coming out of isolation, show persistent difficulties during their adolescence: they play very little, copulate rarely, and do not groom; they still largely avoid social contact. Efforts to alleviate these difficulties have been fruitless. When placed for a year with a mature female chimpanzee who has had abundant experience in rearing her own offspring, the experimental animals show little if any benefit. Similarly, therapeutic trials on various drugs, including tranquilizers and stimulants, were ineffective. The search for conditions under which the disturbances may be overcome will continue.

In some monkey experiments, a remarkable degree of compensation for maternal deprivation has been attained by permitting a modest amount of peer play—on a time scale of minutes per day. In its natural habitat, the same species may play hours per day, rather than minutes. This contrast adds interest to the experimental finding. As we have pointed out in discussing schizophrenia, the developmental potentialities of peer relations deserve much further investigation; they have often been neglected in studies of human development.

What does experimental rearing in total isolation resemble in human situations? It comes closest to cases of drastic neglect, probably not often compatible with a viable human organism—though pediatricians and child psychiatrists do see cases of marked mental and physical retardation due to severe neglect. The components of deprivation are not yet clarified. If isolation-reared monkeys are tested in their home cages, they perform adequately on discrimination-learning tasks.

Partial (rather than total) deprivation-rearing is probably more relevant to human disturbances. In a recent report, the effects of rearing 84 monkeys in a bare wire cage were assessed over several years. These animals could see and hear but not touch other animals; intimate interactions were excluded. These rearing conditions produced several major effects upon adults, such as severe deficiencies in mating behavior; severe deficiencies in maternal behavior, including neglect or abuse of the infant, in those females who did manage to mate and become pregnant; progressively increasing and lasting emotional disturbance (depending on how long the partial isolation continued), especially self-directed aggression; highly fearful responses in females; excessive aggression in males; fearful avoidance of other animals accompanied by occasional outbursts of violence; and serious deficiencies in social behavior but adequate discrimination-learning in the home cage. Opportunity for peer play during partial isolation-rearing results in considerable but not complete compensation for these deficiencies. The presence of relatively complex stimulation objects in the cage, and the opportunity for large swinging movements, also seem to ameliorate the effects of partial isolation-rearing.

In general, the isolation-reared primates are exceedingly fearful and highly prone to violence—toward both themselves and others. Evidently, a great deal of social learning over many years is essential for the constructive channeling of aggressive tendencies and for the development of social behavior that is effective in adaptation.

Just as isolation-rearing experiments have provided a model of psychosis, so interanimal-separation experiments have provided a model of depression. Several investigators have produced depression-like behavior by separating mother and infant. There is reason to believe that similar results could be obtained by separating adult monkeys or apes after they have established strong attachment to each other. Such persistent attachments among primates have increasingly been recognized in field studies in natural habitats.

When mother and infant are separated, a depression-like response is observed in both, though most attention has so far been directed to the infants. They typically show immediate signs of distress, especially in their calling and searching behavior for a day or two after separation. This is followed by greatly decreased activity, much less play than before separation, a huddling posture (similar to many human depressives), and diminished food intake (also a prominent feature of human depression). There are some indications of lasting effects due to brief separation. Infants separated from their mothers for only six days (when they are 32 weeks old) show a proneness to emotional disturbance a year later, though special tests are needed to elicit these responses.

There are striking individual differences in the response to separation. Some get more "depressed" than others. It will be of interest to see whether the monkeys who are highly susceptible differ from other monkeys in biological characteristics, such as brain amines or thyroid function. Experimental manipulation of brain amines by pharmacologic techniques prior to separation is possible. Would the amine-depleted monkey show exceptionally severe behavioral reactions to separation? Similarly, treatment of separation-induced "depression" with antidepressant drugs is an interesting possibility. Thus, the primate separation experiments, like the isolation-rearing experiments, provide models of human disorders in which behavioral and biological linkages can be explored more deeply than would be possible in human subjects. To the extent that these experiments are informative, they will tell us where to look in man for crucial points of vulnerability.

DEVELOPMENT OF
AGGRESSIVE BEHAVIOR

The effects of early hormonal variations upon brain organization and later behavior have constituted one of the exciting scientific frontiers of the past decade. For example, brief treatment of newborn female rats with testosterone (a male sex hormone) results in lifelong abolition of female sex behavior and a tendency toward male patterns of aggressive behavior. During the past few years, such work has been extended to monkeys, utilizing the familiar laboratory species, the rhesus macaque. Investigators from several disciplines have given testosterone to pregnant monkeys, spanning roughly the second quarter of gestation. Though it is difficult to maintain pregnancy under these conditions, they have produced abnormal female offspring with some anatomical and behavioral characteristics of the male type. Their work was based on the earlier finding of sex differences in the behavior of infant monkeys, the males being more aggressive. Reliable behavioral norms have been established, documenting these sex differences in behavior during infancy. Indeed, they appear almost as soon as the infants are capable of any sustained activity. In the testosterone experiments, the social behavior of the untreated female offspring was like that already described for other normal females, but the behavior of the treated females (male sex hormone was given to the mother in pregnancy) much more closely resembled that of males. The masculinized female offspring threatened, initiated play, and engaged in rough-and-tumble play patterns more frequently than did the controls. Like normal males, these masculinized females also withdrew less often from the initiations, threats and approaches of other monkeys. So far, eight such female monkeys exposed to male sex hormone while in the uterus have been observed until they reached adult status. As adults, they have continued to exhibit threatening behavior toward other monkeys, but the other aggressive characteristics have diminished somewhat under the laboratory conditions employed so far.

Recent field studies of primate behavior reveal several characteristics of ground-living, old world monkeys that are pertinent to the present discussion. (1) There is much evidence of rough-and-tumble play among males. Their frequent repetition of such play patterns amounts in fact to a kind of practice of aggressive behavior over several years, from infancy onward. In this way, they develop complex motor skills that utilize their formidable anatomy, including their great canine teeth and massive temporal muscles. (2) There are marked sex differences in anatomy and behavior. The adult males defend the troop and also regulate internal disputes within the group.

Taking the experimental and field observations together, it appears that the male's aggressive predisposition (presumably based on genetic factors mediated by hormonal effects on brain differentiation and muscle growth) is developed through social learning and ultimately put to adaptively significant use. These observations pertain rather generally to complex, old world monkeys and great apes that spend much of their time on the ground, and they may well have significance for the evolution of man. It is at least plausible that basic processes of this sort have continued to operate throughout the long course of human evolution. If some such relation between male sex hormone and aggressive behavior (via early effects on brain development) persists in our own species, how might it work? In view of the enormous dependence of our own species on learning processes, it seems quite unlikely that the early exposure of brain cells to male sex hormone would establish fixed, complex patterns of aggressive behavior for a lifetime. Rather, it seems likely that some more general orientation or temperamental predisposition is influenced by early male hormone, so that aggressive patterns are attractive and readily learned.

Thus, experiments with infrahuman mammals have shown that hormones administered during pregnancy or early in infancy can have striking permanent effects on later behavior. They have also shown that these behavioral effects occur, at least in part, by influencing the interests and preferences of the developing organism. How might this problem be examined in human subjects? The monkey experiments have recently been followed by an investigation of girls who had been exposed to androgens *in utero*. Their developing brains had come into contact during fetal life with chemical compounds similar to the male sex hormone. A total of twenty-two such girls have been studied, mostly in the ten- to twelve-year-old range. Those with striking anatomical abnormalities had undergone surgical correction shortly after birth. With interviews and projective tests, information was obtained from each girl and from at least one parent in each of several behavioral categories. The results indicated that the early-androgenized girls, as contrasted with a control group, tended to be described by self and others as tomboys, to engage in outdoor sports requiring energy and vigor, and to prefer toys ordinarily chosen by boys. This is a provocative study that will require replication. These observations raise an important question and illustrate a line of inquiry that has led from basic research on the biology of sex differentiation to an important human problem. It seems increasingly likely that human biobehavioral studies will be guided by a background of investigation with laboratory animals, involving a conjunction of many techniques—biochemical, neurophysiological, genetic, and behavioral.

Other lines of inquiry have highlighted the great importance of social learning in the development of aggressive behavior. Earlier in this report, we mentioned that monkeys raised in isolation from other monkeys tend to be extraordinarily aggressive, both toward themselves and others. Interestingly, this aggressiveness does not decline spontaneously with the passage of years after the monkeys are brought out of isolation. On the contrary, there is some evidence that this aberrant behavior becomes more pronounced as time passes.

In research with preschool children, a remarkable set of findings has recently highlighted the susceptibility of children to learning aggressive patterns by viewing models who act aggressively. In one experiment, preschool children were exposed to an aggressive model attacking a target object for ten minutes in a laboratory situation, while a control group experienced the same situation without an aggressive model. When the children were tested in the same situation six months later, the former were much more aggressive toward the target object than were the latter. A mere ten-minute exposure apparently enhanced physical aggressiveness in the same situation six months later.

Thus, it appears that biological predispositions to learning aggressive patterns and exposure to specific social learning situations may interact to produce great individual differences in aggressiveness during later life. The extreme variations in human aggressiveness often come to psychiatric attention. For instance, the paranoid reactions constitute one of the most serious problems in psychiatry today, and indeed are a serious social problem since paranoid behavior increases the risk of violence and homicide.

Persons suffering from a paranoid disorder tend to view the world with profound and pervasive distrust through much of their lives. They are likely to suffer episodes of distrust so extreme as to involve gross distortions of reality, such as delusions of persecution. During these psychotic episodes, they often experience delusions of grandeur. Thus, they may attack an imagined tormentor with a feeling of justification in the belief that the attack is a service to mankind. A large proportion of political assassinations and mass murders are carried out during episodes of paranoid psychosis.

Since these disorders are difficult to treat in adult life—and often go unrecognized until after a disastrous event—an important avenue for future research lies in early detection and prompt treatment in childhood. Every effort should be made to take preventive measures based on knowledge of factors that contribute to formation of paranoid personality. Yet very little systematic research has been done on development of paranoid attitudes in childhood. Are there genetic predisposing factors? If so, are they mediated by some abnormality of androgen metabolism in early life? Do chromosomal abnormalities have a role in some cases of antisocial behavior, as a few investigators have lately claimed? Does violent abuse by parental figures in early life predispose a child to a paranoid orientation? What about severe neglect and isolation, similar to that experienced by monkeys in the experiments described above? Here as elsewhere, effective conjunction of biological and psychosocial disciplines—so far rarely achieved—holds great promise for future understanding.

It hardly seems necessary to point out the aggressive tendencies of the human species today. Whatever adaptive functions such behavior may have served in man's evolutionary past, there is serious question about its utility in contemporary society. The risks inherent in such behavior have been greatly amplified within our lifetime. Yet these problems at present attract only a modest amount of attention, even within the behavioral science community. It is difficult to imagine a more important area for scientific research in the future.

STRESS AND HORMONES

Research on stress in man has developed a considerable body of evidence in recent years indicating that the anticipation of personal injury may lead to important changes not only in thought, feeling, and action, but also in endocrine and autonomic processes, and hence in a wide variety of visceral functions. Much work in this field has centered on the changes in adrenocortical functioning that occur in association with emotional distress. Investigators have generally found the adrenal gland to be stimulated via the pituitary gland and the brain, under environmental conditions perceived by a person as threatening to him. Usually such personally threatening conditions elicit clearly detectable emotional distress. In some studies, it has been possible to correlate systematically the extent of emotional distress with adrenal hormone levels in blood and urine, each assessed independently. Work in this field has profited greatly by the development of precise, reliable biochemical methods for measuring hormones and related compounds. Hundreds of persons have been studied in various laboratories under conditions of moderately intense distress. The results are quite consistent, showing a significant elevation of adrenal cortical hormones in both blood and urine compared with the levels recorded under nondistress conditions. Moreover, many of the persons in the distress groups have been studied on repeated occasions, and the elevated adrenal cortical hormone levels have been found to be quite persistent when the distress remained unabated. With relief of distress, substantial declines in these adrenal corticosteroids have been observed. Though the data are less adequate, similar studies relying upon newer biochemical methods for measurement of adrenalin and noradrenalin under conditions of emotional distress have yielded similar results. Thus, it appears likely that emotional distress in man is associated with elevated blood and urinary levels of several adrenal hormones. The elevated levels reflect increased secretory activity by the gland and increased activity of the sympathetic nervous system.

We may summarize several major trends of the evidence on adrenal function under conditions of psychological stress: (1) There is an important set of brain regulatory functions acting upon the adrenal gland, particularly through brain structures primarily in the hypothalamus and secondarily in the limbic system. (2) Elevations in plasma and urinary adrenal compounds are regularly observed under difficult circumstances perceived by the individual as threatening to him. (3) There is a positive correlation between the degree of distress experienced by the individual and the tendency toward hormone elevation. (4) Consistent individual patterns have been observed, both in the range within which each person's adrenal hormone levels fluctuate under ordinary circumstances and in the extent of adrenal response to a difficult, disturbing experience. There are similar observations regarding thyroid function. These findings of consistent individual differences in adrenal cortical and thyroid response to environmental conditions touch on the important problem of differential susceptibility to psychological stress. Clinicians have frequently observed the precipitation and exacerbation of a variety of illnesses in association with emotional crisis—not only psychiatric disorders, but a rather wide range of medical problems. Yet it is abundantly clear that many individuals undergo the common stressful experiences of living without developing such disorders. A number of genetic and environmental factors probably contribute to these individual differences in stress response and hence to differential susceptibility to illness. One promising line of inquiry on this topic grows out of work on human biochemical genetics. This approach relates genetically determined differences in metabolism of hormones to behavior under stress.

That genetic factors exert an important influence on brain and endocrine function as well as on behavior has been known since the turn of the century. In recent years, several interesting avenues of research, utilizing genetic techniques, have been explored. The study of "inborn errors of metabolism" has proven to be especially rewarding. Enzymatic defects in metabolic pathways, with deficiencies of products beyond the block in the pathway and accumulation of intermediate compounds behind the block (like the accumulation of water behind a dam) are characteristically found in inborn errors of metabolism. Several errors of this sort have been found in important endocrine biosynthetic pathways, particularly in regard to hormones of the adrenal cortex and the thyroid. The hormones involved in these genetically determined defects are the same ones known to be important in psychological stress responses. Moreover, these hormones also pass from the general circulation into the brain and may produce neurophysiologic and behavioral effects.

As an example, we call attention to the effects of steroid hormones and their metabolites on brain function and behavior. (The same considerations apply to thyroid hormone; but to avoid excessive complication, we confine this discussion to steroid hormones— that is, those of the adrenal cortex and the sex glands.) There is an interesting possibility that abnormal concentrations of steroids might affect brain function adversely under highly stressful conditions in persons partially deficient in respect to steroid hormone synthesis, transport, or disposal. There is now considerable evidence that a variety of fat-soluble steroids have access to the brain and may produce neurophysiologic, pharmacologic, and behavioral effects. This applies both to hormones, such as cortisol and progesterone, and to some of their closely related metabolites. Progesterone and several of its metabolites are potent anaesthetic agents. 11-Deoxycortisol (which accumulates in one of the genetic blocks of cortisol biosynthesis) is potent in producing convulsions in rats. Indeed, a variety of steroids notably affect seizure thresholds in mammals. Some, like 11-deoxycortisol and cortisol, increase the likelihood of convulsions; while others, like progesterone, decrease it. Recent experiments show marked effects of corticosteroids on somatosensory conduction of nerve impulses from the surface of the body to the hypothalamus and on activity of single nerve cells within that crucial brain region. Given an inborn error of metabolism affecting a steroid pathway, it is quite conceivable that brain function might be adversely affected under stress either by abnormal concentration of the hormone itself (there is considerable clinical evidence of behavioral difficulty in either excess or deficiency of cortisol), or by abnormal concentration of steroids that are metabolites or precursors of cortisol or progesterone. Certain steroid transformations can result in excessive production of toxic metabolites. Further research along these lines promises to yield information significant to clinical medicine.

Some inborn errors of hormone metabolism lead to an excessive production of androgens by the human fetus during pregnancy. This creates a situation similar to those described in the previous section on development of aggressive behavior. As we have indicated, the animal experiments show that during critical periods of development the exposure of the brain to excessive amounts of androgens can produce lasting alterations in sexual and aggressive behavior. It will be an objective of psychiatric research in the next decade to determine what, if any, relevance this basic work has for clinical problems.

Although inborn errors of metabolism tend to be caused by rare genes, and thus the frequency of grossly ill persons having a double dose of the offending gene (homozygotes) is low, heterozygote (single dose) carriers are fairly common. Such individuals may not manifest any obvious evidence of pathology and appear to function adequately under ordinary circumstances. In periods of severe emotional stress, however, continuing excessive demands may be placed on a partially deficient system in such individuals. What happens to persons who have an unusually limited capacity to synthesize adrenocortical or thyroid hormone when they encounter a highly threatening personal situation that is very difficult to resolve? Does a long-term inadequacy of hormone synthesis have detrimental effects on brain function, such that the solution of the precipitating personal problem becomes even more difficult? In pursuit of such questions, an interdisciplinary behavior-endocrine-genetic approach to stress problems offers a promising opportunity for mental health research.

In discussing hormones and stress, we have emphasized those hormones that are best known and most thoroughly studied. Other hormonal products are only now coming under study—for example, the many peptides secreted by the pituitary gland, and compounds such as melatonin from the pineal gland. Present evidence suggests that some of these compounds may affect behavior; more extensive investigation is warranted. In addition, there are hormone-like compounds found endogenously in the brain—neuroregulatory agents, which may function to transmit messages from cell to cell, or as regulators of cell action. Some of these compounds are produced directly in the brain; in all other respects they are identical to the compounds found throughout the body. In response to stress, there is markedly increased production and utilization of some of these compounds. In animals, both severe stress and LSD have the same effects upon some of these brain neuroregulatory agents. More information is needed on the nature of these agents, their functions in the brain, and their role in behavior.

COPING AND ADAPTATION

Psychological responses to stressful experience are central to the work of most psychiatrists. Hence, the literature of psychiatry has provided abundant documentation of the ways in which many common experiences can be traumatic. A variety of situations have been described as threatening and difficult experiences for many individuals. Some of these are inherent components of the life cycle. Others reflect major features of urbanized, industrialized societies. Examples of common stressful experiences that have been emphasized in recent research and clinical discussions are separation from parents in childhood, displacement by siblings, childhood experiences of rejection, illness and injuries of childhood, illness and death of parents, illnesses and injuries of the adult years, the initial transition from home to school, puberty, later school transitions (such as from grade school to junior high school and from high school to college), competitive educational pressures, prolonged graduate education, marriage, pregnancy, menopause, necessity for periodic moves to a new environment, retirement, rapid technological and social change, war and threats of war, and migration.

People vary widely in their responses to such situations. Their appraisal of threat rests heavily on the personal meaning of the situation, which in turn is strongly influenced by a succession of past environments, especially in the family, and by dispositions that have become internalized. The relevance of a given element to motives or values of the person, and conflict among these motives or values, is crucial to the individual's threat appraisal. All this is generally familiar in psychiatry. However, both clinical observation and systematic research have until recently neglected to study the ways in which people cope with the threatening implications of difficult, transitional experiences.

What do we typically do in the face of painful elements of experience? The literature of psychiatry and closely related fields mainly gives the impression that what we do is avoid the painful elements at all costs, reject them as part of ourselves—even if this requires extensive self-deception. The classical mechanisms of defense function largely in this way. Processes such as repression, denial, reaction formation, isolation, and rationalization are centrally concerned with minimizing recognition of potentially distressing aspects of personal experience. They rely heavily upon avoidance and reduction of information.

Is it possible that such mechanisms represent only one important class of responses to threatening elements of experience? Are there other major ways in which the human organism copes with stressful experience? In recent years, there has been increasing recognition of the need to explore these questions. From various disciplines, behavioral scientists have begun to investigate coping, interpersonal problem-solving, and adaptive behavior. For example, a series of studies has explored the ways in which individuals (drawn from a broad range of the general population) cope with difficult circumstances. Some of these studies have dealt with situations of life-threatening illness and injury (such as severe burns, severe poliomyelitis and childhood leukemia). Others have dealt with major psychosocial transitions (such as going away to college, the first pregnancy). These studies of coping behavior have described how people seek and utilize information under stressful conditions.

In difficult circumstances the human organism tends to seek information about several questions: How can the distress be relieved? How can a sense of personal worth be maintained? How can a rewarding continuity of interpersonal relationship be maintained? How can the requirements of the stressful task be met, or the opportunities utilized? Psychological preparation centers on the availability of time to obtain answers to these questions prior to a threatening event. With time, the threatening event can be managed in spite of difficulty; or the blow, if it must come, can be absorbed in the prospect of substitute, alternative sources of self-esteem and rewarding interpersonal relationships. If the threatening event occurs without warning (as in the situation of sudden illness or injury), time for "preparation" is likely to be bought by temporary self-deception. In this way, recognition of threatening elements is made gradual and manageable. A time scale of weeks or a few months for preparation, as in chronic diseases of slow onset, appears to have considerable utility. Where a time scale of many months or even a few years is involved, as in the transitions of youth, exceedingly gradual, thorough, multifaceted preparation is likely to occur.

The threatened person seeks answers to these questions in many ways and from many sources—directly and indirectly, overtly and covertly, in fantasy and in action. Strategies for obtaining and utilizing such information are formed at all levels of awareness and may be employed over long periods of time. Strategies that are established in a person's psychological repertoire, and that have served similar functions in earlier stressful experiences, are likely to be employed first. But distress of high intensity or long duration is a powerful impetus to the formation of new strategies, integrating internalized orientations and current opportunities. Such new strategies, if effective, are likely to become available for use in future crises, and indeed may broaden the individual's problem-solving capacities. But all of us are familiar with unhappier outcomes. What then are the factors that govern the exceedingly diverse outcomes of stressful experience?

Research on the framework of human adaptation is badly needed. We have become experts in diagnosing latent psychopathology, but we have much more to learn about the development of competence, interpersonal problem-solving, and coping behavior under stress. This is another frontier on which psychiatrists are joining with other behavioral scientists in interdisciplinary efforts to clarify important problems.

SLEEP AND DREAMING

At the onset of the twentieth century, Freud explored the content and organization of dreams in rich detail. Indeed, the study of dreams was crucial in his effort to clarify the nature of unconscious mental processes—and thus at the heart of psychoanalytic theory. As psychoanalytic practice spread in the United States, many papers appeared in the professional literature, based on clinical impressions and mainly applying Freud's guidelines for interpreting the personal meaning of an individual's dreams. However, very little systematic research was carried out, and efforts to link the psychology of dreams with the biology of sleep were largely lacking. Then, rather abruptly, a revival of interest in sleep and dreaming occurred, with a broader scientific base for the research.

Since the mid-50s, psychiatrists have joined with scientists of many disciplines in the study of sleep. We were vividly reminded that we spend one-third of our lives in a state about which very little was then known. In the intervening years, the problems of sleep have become one of the major frontiers of science. A new psychobiology of sleep is emerging. From many sides, and in unexpected directions, studies of brain waves, heart rate, breathing, movement, attention, and sleep loss have illuminated puzzling sleep disorders and symptoms of mental illness. Different phases or states of sleep have been delineated, and the brain mechanisms underlying them are now being clarified in some of the most exciting scientific inquiry of our time.

Because the sleeping person appears largely inactive, it had long been assumed that his brain too was resting. This bit of conventional wisdom must now yield to the discovery that the activity of the brain is very lively indeed during one state of sleep. Thus, a night's sleep is typically punctuated by lengthy intervals of fast, low voltage electrical activity of the brain's surface. At the same time, rapid eye movements occur (hence this state is often called REM sleep). Yet the skeletal muscles are completely flaccid during REM sleep. The heart rate and breathing are uneven. When the sleeper is awakened, he usually reports that he has been dreaming. This REM sleep occupies about 20 to 25 percent of a night's sleep—far more dreaming than had generally been assumed to occur.

In contrast, the remainder of a night's sleep is mainly characterized by large, slow waves on the electroencephalogram (EEG), steady heart rate and breathing, and little if any vivid dream recall. This state (sometimes called NREM sleep) is quite different in many ways, physiologically and psychologically, from REM sleep. For example, during REM sleep, electrical activity resembles that of the waking brain; the NREM sleep waves do not.

These differences in the two kinds of sleep have been confirmed by newer techniques measuring the electrical activity of single brain cells in experimental animals during different states of sleep and wakefulness. When micro-electrodes are used to record from single brain cells in the visual cortex, the average discharge frequency is about twice as high during REM sleep as during NREM sleep. Indeed, the frequency during REM sleep is equal to that of the waking animal paying close attention to its environment. High levels of electrical activity during REM sleep have also been observed with micro-electrode measurements in various other parts of the brain. Other measurements of brain activity, such as oxygen consumption and blood flow, also show elevated levels during REM sleep. All mammals so far studied (and this includes many different species) show REM sleep. So perhaps we are not the only dreaming animal; at any rate, the physiologic basis of dreaming is widely present.

Scientists have combined neurophysiological, biochemical and behavioral techniques to locate sleep-inducing brain cells and find out how they work. One crucial collection of nerve cells at the midline of the brainstem, known as raphé cells, is currently the object of much experimental attention. Under ultraviolet light, these cells emit a yellow fluorescence, indicating that they contain the hormone-like substance, serotonin. This neuroregulatory agent has been implicated in brain function by several lines of inquiry. Drug and brain lesion studies indicated that it might have a role in sleep. For example, injections of a chemical compound (5-hydroxytryptophan) that produces elevation of brain serotonin elicit more NREM sleep and less REM sleep.

Interesting further information about the role of serotonin in sleep has come from studies using cats in which chemical inhibitors of serotonin formation have been given to animals. At first there is a cessation of sleep and REM sleep. After a few days of continued administration of inhibitors of serotonin synthesis, sleep returns almost to normal. However, there is a profound disturbance in REM sleep. The events of REM sleep called "phasic events" (including such characteristics as eye movements and electrical spikes from some areas of the brain, called PGO spikes) move from the REM period to the waking state and the non-REM sleep state. In addition, animals treated chronically with inhibitors of serotonin formation develop very bizarre behavior.

The evidence accumulated thus far would suggest that, at least in the cat, serotonin has a role in sleep and that after serotonin formation is inhibited for about a week adaptive processes may develop that allow a return of sleep, either through the formation of very small amounts of serotonin or by some mechanism as yet unclarified. However, the return to sleep is not accompanied by a return to normal REM periods, and bizzare behavior is noted in the animals. Further, it has been demonstrated that in rats deprived of REM sleep there is an increased turnover in the formation and utilization of serotonin.

In related research, it has been found that cats chronically given a compound that inhibits serotonin formation do not have a rebound of REM sleep after deprivation of REM sleep, in contrast to all other situations in which, after REM deprivation, the animal normally makes up REM sleep on a quite exact basis. Of interest is the finding that some schizophrenic patients, when deprived of REM sleep, also do not make up REM sleep later. These findings have led to the speculation that the animal deprived chronically of serotonin is a model system in which there may be an analogy to the schizophrenic situation; in both the currently ill schizophrenic patient and in these animals the events of REM sleep may be occurring during the waking state. This view is consistent with the psychoanalytic observation of similarity between dreams and psychotic experiences. Further investigation is necessary to determine whether in the human serotonin or some other neuroregulatory agent may be involved in normally separating the events of REM sleep from the waking state, and whether such a compound may be relevant to the control of the phasic events of REM sleep.

The neural basis of REM sleep is also under investigation. By making lesions systematically in various parts of the brain of experimental animals, crucial cell clusters have been specified. REM sleep can be abolished by destroying nerve cells in a portion of the pons known as the locus coeruleus. Histochemical techniques have shown that these cells contain noradrenalin. Quite possibly, noradrenalin plays a role in mediating REM sleep similar to that of serotonin in NREM sleep.

This research moves us toward an understanding of the brain mechanisms underlying dreaming. The controlling cells apparently are located in the pons. The firing of these cells sends messages mainly to the brain's visual tracts; presumably these are important in the visual imagery of dreaming. But even when these cells are strongly stimulated, the body's motor system remains inactive during sleep; there is a powerful inhibition of movement. If the locus coeruleus is experimentally destroyed, the animal periodically exhibits bursts of activity, which suggest to observers the hallucinations of a dream. At such times, the animal shows all the signs of REM sleep except that it exhibits bodily movements of rage, fear, or pursuit, sustained sometimes for several minutes. The long-term effects of such lesions are not yet clear.

While the new biology of sleep has been advancing so remarkably, there have not yet been comparable rapid advances in the psychology of dreaming. When REM sleep was discovered, the possibility immediately arose of obtaining access to a far larger sample of dream activity than had ever been available before—and with less time intervening between the dream and its report. Freud had relied heavily on dream interpretation in building his system of depth psychology. He had emphasized the disguised wish-fulfillment function of dream; dreams reflected fundamental, personal motivations. Some later psychoanalysts broadened this concept by calling attention to problem-solving implications of dream content. For example, dreams of men in combat sometimes reworked a disturbing experience until it came out with a more acceptable ending. Some psychoanalysts examined dreams in close detail for therapeutic purposes, attempting to detect in dreams personally threatening implications in a day's events, their meaning for the individual, and his efforts to cope with them. Viewed in this way, the newer sleep laboratories might provide useful tools for the study of human motivation and coping behavior. But so far this tradition has generated little systematic research, let alone experimental approaches. The great bulk of experimental effort has gone into variables that are easier to measure and control. Still some inklings of future investigation of dream content have appeared, and others come to mind. Among the approaches that hold promise are the presentation of problematic or disturbing material to subjects just before they go to sleep; the identification of conspicuous characteristics of laboratory personnel that could be traced in dream content, following the sequence of a given theme through a night's dreams; comparison of the report of a given dream during the night with its report in the morning; comparison of dream contents in stressful and nonstressful periods of the subject's life; testing the effects of drugs and hormones, such as adrenalin, on dream content.

Another way of viewing dreaming—not necessarily in conflict with that described above—has arisen in the past few years. This view rests on an analogy between brain and computer. Such analogies have been stimulating in other contexts and deserve attention here. Mammalian brains have two general forms of memory storage—short-term and long-term. Events a person has experienced are first recorded in a labile system that has a high storage capacity but a short life. This system probably rests on electrical arrangements and does not require protein synthesis in the brain. Over time, these events are accepted or rejected for long-term storage according to built-in criteria, some of which have been established in the lifetime of the individual and therefore reflect his distinctive outlook. Presumably, events relevant to the person's enduring motivations are useful in guiding his behavior and are therefore transferred to permanent memory storage. Recent work in experimental animals has shown that this process requires protein synthesis in the brain. Thus, scanning of the material in short-term memory storage must occur to permit useful selection and classification for long-term storage.

Similar processes are now commonplace in computer technology. Periodically, computer programs must be revised and reclassified to keep them up to date. To do this, the computer must be taken temporarily offline, that is, uncoupled from its regular tasks. In this analogy, the brain is offline during sleep, with action tendencies inhibited, and so is free to review its programs and update them. Dreaming is considered the psychological reflection of this process. One of the interesting ramifications of this analogy is developmental. Computer programs are most likely to require modification when there is a large input of new information. In early life, when new experiences are most voluminous, the organism requires more sleep and a larger proportion of it is REM (dreaming) sleep. Perhaps these observations have a functional relation. In any event, it may be anticipated that the next decade will see many efforts to explore the utility of computer models for brain function and behavior.

The investigation of hormones in relation to the new biology of sleep has drawn less attention than might reasonably have been expected. However, a recent surprising finding deserves interest. It has been discovered that human growth hormone is secreted in rather large amounts during sleep. Moreover, the release of this hormone seems linked rather specifically to slow-wave, NREM, deep sleep. When healthy human subjects abruptly changed their sleep-waking cycle by twelve hours (similar to a worker changing from a day shift to a night shift), the release of growth hormone with sleep was reversed. It has been suggested that this release of growth hormone is part of a set of restorative physiological processes in slow-wave sleep and is under the control of neuroendocrine circuits located deep in the brain. (See also the section, Stress and Hormones.)

Several laboratories have been exploring the behavioral and physiological consequences of repeated and/or prolonged deprivation of REM sleep, and the neurophysiological and neurochemical mechanisms through which REM-deprivation effects occur. One major finding is perhaps reminiscent of Freud's view of dreaming; experimental animals deprived of REM sleep for long periods (though not deprived of total sleep time) show heightened motivation in several spheres crucial for species survival. Their motivation for eating, sexual activity, and aggressive behavior becomes very intense. There is some evidence that human subjects may eventually become disturbed under these conditions, but ethical considerations have limited experimental research on this problem. However, systematic study of naturally occurring sleep-deprivation may help to clarify this problem.

In any event, it has been shown that the REM portion of sleep may be specifically diminished by a variety of means: several drugs that affect the brain; episodes of intense anxiety; experimental awakenings. No matter how REM sleep is diminished, normal individuals make up for this loss as soon as they are permitted to sleep undisturbed; that is, there is a compensatory rebound in REM time following REM deprivation. This well-confirmed fact suggests some sort of biological need for a quota of REM sleep. Two interesting exceptions to this compensatory rebound after REM deprivation have recently been discovered (and are referred to above). One occurs when experimental animals undergo depletion of brain serotonin; the other exists in currently ill schizophrenic patients. This observation has done much to enhance interest in the clinical implications of sleep research.

This brings us to questions regarding sleep loss in general. Psychiatrists have been active in interdisciplinary research on the possible consequences of sleep loss, as in other areas of sleep research. As evidence has accumulated, especially from systematic studies, it has become apparent that sleep deprivation leads to intermittent gaps in performance ("lapses"); these lapses increase in frequency and severity with increasing sleep loss. Differential loss of REM sleep, in addition to the effects mentioned above, may specifically diminish the ability to maintain vigilance. It may also underlie the irritability of sleep loss. Differential loss of slow-wave sleep, on the other hand, may specifically impair ability to carry out numerical calculation. Many investigators anticipate that different states of sleep will in time be shown to serve different restorative functions. By the same token, differential deprivation may turn out to have different clinical consequences.

In any event, when total sleep time is sharply restricted for days on end, severe disturbances are likely to occur. The person tends to suffer sensory disorders—illusions of visual and tactile sensation that may even develop into hallucinations. Lapses of attention (microsleep intervals) become very frequent. There is a tendency to withdraw from activity, to become disoriented in time, place, and person. The extent of the effects are influenced by many environmental factors and by the subject's motivation. Unstable distrustful persons may be especially vulnerable. Young people seem more resistant to prolonged sleep-deprivation. A characteristic effect of sleep loss is the slowing of the waking alpha rhythm shown by the electroencephalogram (EEG). Stress hormones in the blood tend to show a modest elevation early in sleep loss; biochemical changes often occur within 48 hours. Changes in energy metabolism have been the object of some investigation, particularly the question whether they might be related to the psychotic symptoms that are likely to occur after about 120 hours of sleep-deprivation. This is an area for future behavioral-biochemical research.

A single night of uninterrupted sleep appears to minimize these symptoms; yet there are beginning to be indications that repeated episodes of sleep disturbance, as occur so often in the insomnia of acute emotional distress, may have some lasting effects. This is an important area for clinical investigation. Regarding this problem, as elsewhere in sleep research (such as research on the effects of drugs), it has been very profitable to move back and forth between observations of experimental animals and human subjects, including psychiatric patients.

The clinical relevance of sleep research is already apparent. Some surprises have emerged, and others are likely to appear in the near future. Narcolepsy, a disorder characterized by frequent lapses into sleep during the day, even in the midst of ongoing activities, is being clarified. The daytime sleep lapses are primarily bursts of REM sleep. Some narcoleptics have a long history of chaotic sleep patterns associated with severe family problems. Evidently they are markedly REM-deprived at night and tend to compensate inadvertently during the day. Treatment of this disorder has improved since the discovery of its REM character.

Heart attacks, often fatal, are peculiarly likely to occur in the early morning hours when most REM sleep is concentrated. The possible bearing of sleep physiology upon coronary circulation deserves investigation in light of this fact, and the finding that attacks of nocturnal pain in patients with coronary heart disease occur primarily during REM periods.

Currently, psychiatric research workers are especially interested in clarifying the sleep disorders of depressions and schizophrenia. In several laboratories, a substantial number of these patients have now been studied, including various subgroups. The depression research serves well to illustrate an exciting line of inquiry in clinical psychobiology. A series of depressed patients has been studied in detail, with all-night EEG sleep recordings made in the patient's own bed in a familiar hospital situation. At first these studies were cross-sectional; more recently, they have been longitudinal, utilizing nightly recordings from one to seven months in various patients. The EEG sleep recordings can be compared with systematic sleep observations made by the nursing staff, and with daily clinical ratings made independently by the ward staff during daytime hours. The most useful comparisons involve three groups: psychotic depressives; neurotic depressives; and age-matched control subjects.

We can only briefly summarize the main findings of these studies.

In the normal person, there is remarkable consistency in the overall patterning of sleep through the night, even though details vary from person to person and from night to night for each individual. Most studies have been done on young adults. Recent work on older people shows changes with age. With the passage of years, the continuity of sleep tends to be increasingly broken by transient awakenings; the proportion of deep sleep (as measured by EEG patterns) decreases; and the total amount of sleep decreases.

In depressed patients, the most striking sleep abnormalities are shown by those who are clearly psychotic. In general, the more severe the depression, the greater is the tendency toward sleep abnormalities. Psychotic depressive patients show marked fragmentation and shallowness of sleep. EEG patterns rarely go beyond the most superficial stages of sleep; the deepest sleep ("stage four" sleep) is greatly diminished. There are many awakenings through the night. Unlike normal persons and even unlike the moderately depressed, these patients go into REM periods very soon after falling asleep. The eye movements during sleep are exceptionally intense. REM periods frequently appear at unusually short intervals. There is extreme variability among these psychotic depressives in the percentage of sleep time occupied by REM sleep. The total duration of sleep is very low.

When emotional turmoil is very intense, REM sleep tends to be greatly diminished. This is not specific to severe depression, since similar measurements have been made in acutely schizophrenic patients and in tensely anxious patients. Evidently REM is especially vulnerable to intense emotional distress, and this vulnerability may occur in various diagnostic entities. So, in effect, the patient in great distress becomes REM-deprived. As mentioned earlier, one of the most remarkable discoveries in sleep research has been the REM rebound that occurs after REM deprivation. It is as though there is a pressure for REM expression that builds up whenever REM is suppressed in some way. This pressure is manifested in several ways: (1) REM periods occur very shortly after falling asleep. (2) There are increasingly frequent REM periods through the night. (3) In animal studies of prolonged REM deprivation, there is an extraordinary intensity of the REM phasic events, including the eye movements. This is the very constellation that occurs so strikingly in the psychotic depressives. Therefore, the question has been raised whether these persons have undergone prolonged, severe REM deprivation as a consequence of prolonged emotional disturbance. Moreover, these severe depressions are most likely to occur at an age when sleep is more susceptible to disruption than in youth. So, some investigators are exploring a model built on the following general sequence: loss, grief, or other adverse environmental event; prolonged emotional distress; diminution of total sleep time, and especially of REM sleep; exceptional individual vulnerability to sleep disruption; effects of sleep disturbance further interfere with person's ability to cope with personal and environmental problems. Such a model might well have relevance not only for depression but for schizophrenia as well.

Recent work with schizophrenic patients shows clearly that sleep characteristics are different in different phases of the illness. Here as elsewhere, broad diagnostic categories (such as schizophrenia and depression) are inadequate for refined analysis of research problems. In any event, the pervasive and profound sleep disturbances of mental illness are now becoming the object of major interdisciplinary study, linking behavioral, neurophysiological, and biochemical measures. In view of the impressive individual differences noted in almost every phase of sleep research, it is surprising that little attention has so far been given to genetic factors. Perhaps the approach of human biochemical genetics will be helpful here, as with stress research. Also, closer collaboration between physiological and psychological investigators should prove rewarding.

5

TOWARD THE SOLUTION OF PSYCHIATRIC PROBLEMS

In this closing chapter, we will discuss general topics that cut across the length and breadth of this book. We hope that the preceding substance of the book will make our recommendations meaningful. They will, of course, have different utility for readers in different positions. Some of our recommendations are intended mainly for units of government, some for students, and some for the scientific community. There are also recommendations intended for private foundations, for professional organizations, for universities, and for the general public. Most recommendations are relevant to more than one group. For the most part, we wish to make general comments that will help clarify the current position of the field and its prospects for future improvement. These comments often contain implicit or explicit recommendations, of a "to whom it may concern" character. We hope that each reader will consider each point in the context of his own interests and opportunities, wearing the shoe if it fits.

SOLUTION OF PSYCHIATRIC PROBLEMS: MATTERS OF CONCERN

In keeping with the original impetus for this series of books provided by the National Academy of Science and the Social Science Research Council, we have discussed psychiatry as a behavioral science. We have dealt with the service and educational

81

aspects of the field only insofar as they are directly relevant to its scientific base. We have tried to point out promising directions of research in several scientific disciplines bearing directly on problems of human suffering, for which psychiatry has great responsibility. We have emphasized the social responsibilities and the scientific opportunities facing the field. In so doing, we have called attention to facets of psychiatry that have not been widely known or deeply understood.

Along the way, we have pointed out many shortcomings, limitations, and unsolved problems. Now we ask ourselves, Are there matters of general concern regarding the future progress of the field? While many obstacles have been overcome, what obstacles remain which might seriously interfere with solution of the terribly important problems faced by psychiatry and its closely related fields?

Efforts to strengthen the scientific aspects of psychiatry have certainly encountered difficulties. Within the field, many clinicians have been suspicious of science, for a variety of reasons. Some have felt that the important answers were already available. Others believed that scientific method could not be applied to human behavior, however desirable it might be to do so. Some have been concerned that the field might change too rapidly.

Indeed, at an earlier time, the field was characterized by intense differences of opinion (and much bitterness) among conflicting "schools," each of which tended to be quite dogmatic and impermeable to new evidence. Most schools claimed a scientific mantle for their positions. The orientation of these schools toward students and practitioners implied an all-or-none attitude, something like, "You're either for us or against us."

These difficulties within the field have greatly diminished in recent years. But they have left their mark, both within and outside the field. A large proportion of today's practicing psychiatrists were trained in an era when there was not a strong scientific orientation in the field, and indeed no strong expectation of future change in the field, whatever its source. This is true also of those working in university settings. Thus, the recent shift toward an expectation of new developments and a greater appreciation of the relevance of science for psychiatry has necessarily been viewed with mixed feelings.

For a variety of reasons, prominently including the field's internal difficulties, the scientific community has viewed psychiatry with some suspicion, and at the same time with considerable interest. The level

is report would have been impossible without NIMH
a tiny beginning about two decades ago, NIMH has
me a large agency. This reflects vigorous leadership
titute. It also reflects a high degree of congressional,
id public support. Indeed, a plausible argument can
he urgent importance of the problems tackled by psy-
ated disciplines was recognized more rapidly by the
and its elected representatives than by the medical
ommunities. In any event, NIMH now provides major
ly for research but also for education and for mental

en deep concern in the scientific community in recent
Institute's research support might become dangerously
ie face of tight budgets and a rapidly growing com-
vice programs. Here as elsewhere in medicine, there
rences of opinion concerning the extent to which prog-
de simply by applying present knowledge to clinical
ie mental health field, with its short tradition of sci-
is particularly important that new knowledge be gen-
y through direct study of clinical problems but also
esearch on the fundamental nature of behavior.
ical field, progress depends on a balance between at-
problems of contemporary patients and patients of fu-
s. This involves complex judgments about which ef-
o yield prompt benefit for current patients, and which
at promise that can only be fulfilled with long-range
dgments affect allocation of resources at every level of
l private activity.
he National Institute of Mental Health, government
enerally been quite ambivalent toward psychiatry and
behavioral sciences. They have, for the most part, been
ike up the challenge or recognize the opportunity.
e past few years have notable signs of improvement
National Institute of Child Health and Human De-
taken some encouraging initial steps toward support
development of behavior. The National Institute of
l Sciences has made a modest beginning in support
oral science. The National Institute of Neurological
troke has supported brain research pertinent to be-
tional Heart Institute has sometimes shown interest

of awareness of newer scier
report, has not been high.
terms either of the most ir
pits") or in terms of the p
a doctrinaire caricature). T
sity of research approaches
gone largely unappreciated

The ambivalence of th
has been manifested in dif
tists and clinical investigat
been highly critical of p
promising scientific efforts
major scientific prizes and
to work on psychiatric pro
member of the National .
been active in the Natio:
ever served on the Presic
very few have participated
tradition of psychiatry, an
no doubt accounts for mu
So also does the inheren
matter. But these factors :
the old prescientific uneas
the most intimate matter
with the situation. Morec
of conventional wisdom
is his own expert. Yet the
more urgent than ever. I
has had a hard row to ho
and scientific communit
this struggle is being wo
recent and no one can ye
useful to understand the
had to develop their work

In the last analysis, th
the promise of psychiat
quate financial support
the main source of such
Mental Health (NIMH
Education, and Welfare

described in t
support. Fron
grown to bec
within the In
presidential, a
be made that
chiatry and r
general publi
and scientific
support not o
health services

There has b
years that the
restricted in t
mitment to s
have been diff
ress can be m
problems. In
entific work, i
erated, not on
through basic

In every cli
tention to the
ture generatio
forts are likely
efforts offer gr
effort. These j
government an

Apart from
agencies have
closely related
very slow to t
Only within t
occurred. The
velopment has
of research on
General Medi
of basic behav
Diseases and
havior. The N

in behavioral problems pertinent to cardiovascular disorders. There is an appreciable risk that the current tight federal budget will induce these institutes to back away from their explorations in behavioral science. We need hardly add in the context of this book that such a retreat would be a serious error. On the contrary, we hope that this book, along with the others in this Behavioral and Social Science series, makes it evident why a greater commitment to behavioral science by the National Institutes of Health would be highly desirable.

In this connection, the increased recognition of the behavioral sciences and increased support provided by the National Science Foundation have been heartening developments. However, support for further development of behavioral science by the NSF is now in jeopardy because of the exceptionally heavy budgetary pressure to which the Foundation has lately been subjected. Should the support of basic behavioral science falter, the underpinning for ultimate solution of psychiatric problems would be gravely damaged.

Since the fifty state governments within the United States have so much responsibility for care of the mentally ill, some states have shown interest in supporting research. In most states, such support has been sharply restricted or nonexistent. But a few states have had the vision to build research institutes, usually in conjunction with one or more universities. This commendable development has moved slowly, chiefly because well-trained research personnel have been in terribly short supply. Very few states have made significant funds available to private institutions within their borders, even when these have had unusual capability for conducting research on the very problems that constitute such a burden for the states.

Within psychiatry itself, there are still only a few university departments of outstanding scientific caliber. Curiously, the universities were slow to provide intellectual leadership in this field. In the great period of psychiatric growth following World War II, the departments of psychiatry served mainly as preparatory schools for psychoanalytic institutes, which were heavily committed to private practice of a narrow-spectrum specialty rather than to generating new information or clinical innovations. In the next two sections, we sketch some promising recent developments, including the emergence of a new breed of university department—and make suggestions for further improvement.

RELATION OF PSYCHIATRY
TO OTHER SCIENTIFIC DISCIPLINES

The scientific aspects of psychiatry present formidable difficulties, but they also present unusual stimulation and opportunity. Psychiatry sits at the point of conjunction between the biological and behavioral sciences. It is faced with problems of great practical importance and entrusted with substantial public responsibility. By now, it is clear that serious disorders of behavior may arise from many influences—biological, psychological, and social. Hence, many kinds of skills are required to make reasonable headway toward clarifying, dealing with, and ultimately preventing various sources of human suffering. Moreover, there is much in psychiatry's medical heritage that is oriented toward following whatever evidence may be relevant to disease and distress. Given public trust in the physician, the psychiatrist is in an unusually favorable position to explore even the most intimately personal matters. The situation is in a way analogous to the role of early biomedical research workers in examining urine, feces, and the bodies of deceased persons. The physician has long been exempted from taboos that confine other investigators, and has tacit social permission to trespass into areas otherwise off limits, as long as his behavior is ethical and serves the patient's welfare. This gives him access to information less likely to be available to others.

Newer possibilities for generating psychiatric information of greater dependability and penetration have emerged in recent years from biological and psychosocial disciplines. Almost every discipline in the biological and behavioral sciences has some aspect that is directly relevant to psychiatric problems. Such relevance is clearly apparent in biological fields—biochemistry, neurophysiology, genetics, and evolution. There is a behavioral aspect to each of these disciplines. In the psychological fields, the early preoccupation of psychiatry with clinical psychology has been broadened to include great interest in other areas, such as developmental psychology, motivation and learning, normal personality, and social psychology. The attention paid to rigorous methods in psychological disciplines has recently had a strong impact on psychiatric research. With respect to sociology and anthropology, psychiatric interest has risen dramatically during the past decade in such subfields as epidemiology, cross-cultural research, the study of behavior in large organizations, sociobiology, and especially the family and other small groups. Thus the unique opportunity of psychiatric research is the establishment of certain vital linkages between biological, psychological, and social sciences; and between the clinical and basic aspects of each. A few university departments of psychiatry now have on their faculties people from each of these various backgrounds. Psychiatry in its scientific aspects has begun to stimulate diverse groups in the scientific community, and to provide a context for some integration of diverse contributions. Perhaps psychiatry will be able to contribute to the emergence of a broader concept of the life sciences, one that includes biology and behavior.

Among the disciplines concerned with living organisms, the need for communication is nowhere more apparent than in the study of psychiatric problems. Yet such communication is not easily achieved. Indeed, the early interdisciplinary ventures proved so difficult that it became fashionable to deride such efforts. Tensions and stereotypes, partly derived from older difficulties in PhD-MD relations, have interfered. Traditionally, scientists with PhDs have tended to view physicians as poorly prepared for scientific work and overly preoccupied with status and power. PhDs have been concerned with their low status in medical school faculties—though their status has risen dramatically in recent years. On the other hand, physicians have had traditional misgivings about scientists with PhDs. In an earlier time, practicing physicians tended to view them as impractical, highly abstract, far removed from the firing line of clinical practice. Physicians in full-time academic work have zealously guarded their high status derived from medical qualifications. So the effective incorporation of outstanding basic scientists into medical school faculties has been a gradual process, extending over about half a century. The advent of behavioral scientists on these faculties is the newest step in this process, and hence the one least well established. Moreover, in the fields concerned with human behavior, there has been a traditional tension over the issue of precision versus relevance. Clinicians have tended to view basic scientists as being overly occupied with a facade of scientific respectability, measuring with great precision variables of trivial significance. Conversely, basic scientists have tended to view clinical investigators as messy, dealing with potentially important variables so sloppily that results could hardly be reproducible. In our judgment, these tensions and barriers to communication have greatly diminished in the past decade, though much remains to be done. At least the groundwork for effective communication and co-operation has been established.

The time is ripe for enhancement of the current trend toward appointment of behavioral scientists to medical school faculties. It is already apparent that behavioral scientists from many disciplines have an important place in departments of psychiatry. They are now beginning to appear in other medical school departments—pediatrics, internal medicine, preventive medicine, and some basic science departments. Indeed, a few medical schools have established new departments in the behavioral sciences. Behavioral scientists are increasingly appearing on the faculties of schools of public health. Some of the most productive research on problems of behavior has been carried out in medically oriented research institutions such as the National Institute of Mental Health (in its intramural program), the Walter Reed Army Institute of Research, and the Rockefeller University.

In view of the wide range of competence required for effective psychiatric research, there is a need to strengthen and diversify research programs throughout the country. This may be done in several ways. One is by providing attractive conditions that will bring specialists from other disciplines into departments of psychiatry. This has already been done to some extent in attracting psychologists. Beyond this, the process is in an early stage of development, but a few psychiatry departments have shown that excellent scientists of various backgrounds may be recruited into psychiatric units and work effectively there. The survey of professional schools conducted as part of the present Behavioral and Social Science Survey revealed that the responding schools of medicine have appointed 377 psychologists and 84 sociologists. These data are reported in *The Behavioral and Social Sciences: Outlook and Needs* (Englewood Cliffs, N.J.: Prentice-Hall, 1969). Beyond these two fields, however, the behavioral sciences are sparsely represented: indeed, no responding school has an economist on its faculty, despite the clear relevance of economics to contemporary problems of medical care. The compelling implication of these survey responses is the need for additional *diversity* in behavioral science competence in medical school faculties; and this need is certainly not limited to departments of psychiatry.

A second approach involves collaboration of psychiatrists with specialists working in other departments. There are notable instances of the success of this approach, but such interdepartmental ventures are still uncommon. The traditional insularity of psychiatry from other fields of medicine and science has been a handicap, but one that is now being overcome.

A third approach, long employed in other fields of medicine, such as internal medicine, pediatrics and surgery, is to send young specialists to work for a time in a basic science field so that new skills may be learned and then be applied to clinical problems. Psychiatry has been slow to take up this practice, but instances of it are now appearing. We believe it to be a particularly promising avenue for developing psychiatry as a science. It will permit academic psychiatry to draw on the scientific strengths of the biological and psychosocial disciplines. These strengths might be brought into psychiatry in several ways: by recruiting for psychiatry individuals who have had a strong scientific background prior to studying medicine; by utilizing the elective time in the medical school years for basic science research training; by offering a research fellowship immediately after the clinical internship, before the physician enters the psychiatric residency; by expanding the elective time during residency training and arranging for use of this time in research training; and by postresidency research fellowships. These possibilities are not mutually exclusive. The basic point is that there are a variety of ways in which young psychiatrists, and psychiatrists-to-be, can acquire substantial strength in basic science which can then be applied to clinical problems. This blending of basic and clinical skills in certain gifted, dedicated individuals can be of great benefit for the field. University departments of psychiatry may need to provide a "heat shield" for the period of reentry—the time in which the clinician-scientist is working out the practical, day-to-day integration of the two major streams of his experience. This responsibility will rest mainly on departmental chairmen, and can only be done effectively on a highly individualized basis. There is little precedent for this new breed of psychiatric scientist. In another decade, the patterns of their career development should be well established.

The current trend in medical education toward increasing individuality, flexibility in curriculum, and more elective time, provides the opportunity for medical students and psychiatric residents to do graduate work in behavioral science departments. Such arrangements can be of mutual benefit to the fields concerned. For example, students in the behavioral sciences can work in psychiatry departments, getting supervised clinical experience, participating in research and clinical conferences, and conducting thesis research. Indeed, we are generally impressed with the stimulus that psychiatric problems can provide for scientists and students in other fields. Therefore, we recommend that universities greatly increase opportunities for access to psychiatric research and, with adequate safeguards, to clinical situations.

Another way to link psychiatry with other behavioral science disciplines is through interdisciplinary training programs, such as the biology and behavior training program of the National Institute of Mental Health. Such a training program requires an interdisciplinary (and usually interdepartmental) faculty. It also typically involves the mixing of students from various fields. Thus, an unusual sharing of information and ideas can be achieved. The NIMH training program in biological sciences pertinent to behavior provides an excellent model for two similar efforts.

First, we recommend strong support for the newly emerging effort of the National Institute of Mental Health to develop an interdisciplinary, research training program in social sciences pertinent to psychiatric problems. These programs should involve long-term collaboration between departments of psychiatry, sociology, anthropology, social psychology, and statistics.

Second, the time has come to mount comprehensive research training programs centering on the *development* of behavior. As we noted in describing promising lines of research, both biological and behavioral sciences are moving strongly on developmental problems. This is a subject of keen interest to undergraduates as well as to graduate students. Universities should meet this interest by undertaking biobehavioral science training programs on development. In medical schools, this might well include participation by departments of psychiatry and pediatrics. In the nonmedical basic sciences, this might include psychology, biology, and social science. Such programs are especially timely in view of growing concern about the effect of early environment on later behavior, and the health problems of children and adolescents. These issues often generate much controversy and little solid information. There is a pressing need for the expansion of the amount of dependable research as a foundation for rational public policy. If such training programs are to move rapidly enough to meet the need, they will require specific recognition and funding from federal agencies and private foundations. The cost is likely to be small in proportion to the potential yield.

It would be helpful if a journal existed specifically for communication of behavioral science research to psychiatry. Such a journal might emphasize review and analysis of major lines of inquiry in behavioral science pertinent to psychiatric problems. Existing journals might be encouraged to include material of this sort, as a new service. In the same vein, joint seminars between psychiatry departments and other behavioral science departments are desirable. At the present time, these are rarely undertaken even on an ad hoc basis. The possibility of regular joint seminars deserves exploration. It would be useful for a group of behavioral science departments in major universities, including psychiatry departments, to organize a "current frontiers" series for workers in other disciplines. On a rotating basis, each discipline would undertake the presentation of certain of its major lines of inquiry in a way that would be aimed not at the technical specialists closest to the work, but rather at those some distance away in related fields. Such presentations at the Center for Advanced Study in the Behavioral Sciences have typically been quite stimulating and have sometimes led to important cross-fertilization in research.

Much experience attests to the value of multidisciplinary environments. Such environments tend to be exceptionally informative. In the long run, they held much promise for the understanding of behavior. Our emphasis here is on multidisciplinary environments rather than on multidisciplinary research. We are emphasizing the potential for members of the various disciplines to learn from each other, and also the potential for mutual technical aid and the opportunity for collaboration. But we are not recommending grand interdisciplinary collaboration. Rather, collaborations may arise spontaneously, given favorable conditions in multidisciplinary environments. It is easy for disciplines to withdraw into functional isolation. However, some factors can help overcome the risks of regimentation and the centrifugal tendencies and failures in communication so familiar in interdisciplinary enterprises. One of these is geographic proximity, which favors frequent, enduring, informal contacts and opportunity for people of different backgrounds to know each other as human beings. Some interdisciplinary groups have also found it useful to set up special seminars on a regular basis that are specifically designed for communication across disciplinary barriers. Publications like *Scientific American* provide useful models for such communication. In some departments, periodic retreats have been useful, concentrating on topics of shared interest for one to several days in pleasant surroundings with careful preparation. Such occasions are useful not only in exchanging information but also in forming personal relationships that favor mutual respect. Where disciplines with very different traditions are involved, time is required for each to learn the essential language, style, and substance of the other, so that communication around a shared interest can be based on understanding and respect.

In the report, *The Behavioral and Social Sciences: Outlook and Needs,* prepared under the auspices of the National Academy of Sciences and the Social Science Research Council, one of the major recommendations is the creation by some universities of graduate schools of applied behavioral science. These would be interdisciplinary schools oriented toward research on persistent social problems. We hope that this recommendation will receive prompt and thorough consideration. When it is implemented—especially at universities where medical schools are on the main campus with the rest of the university—we urge that psychiatry participate vigorously from the start.

SOME CONDITIONS FAVORING EFFECTIVE PSYCHIATRIC RESEARCH

Psychiatry departments have not usually been planned in a way that promotes strong scientific development. The tendency has been to think of psychiatry as a strictly clinical field, with little research activity and no laboratories. There is an urgent need for the provision of adequate laboratory space in psychiatry departments, if research programs are to flourish. Such space should be on a scale comparable to that in departments of medicine, pediatrics, and surgery. Similarly, there is a need for additional full-time positions in most departments. Appointments should be flexible, so as to encourage interdisciplinary research.

More appointments of behavioral and social scientists are needed in a variety of health settings, such as medical schools, schools of public health, neighborhood health centers, and community mental health centers. The behavioral and social science disciplines should be woven into the fabric of health services, education, and research so that they can take advantage of new opportunities to generate information and ideas on human behavior and its disorders.

In this connection, one particularly interesting prospect is the emergence of departments of behavior in schools of medicine. Ideally, these would tend to function as basic science departments, parallel with such departments as physiology and biochemistry. In the past, it has been rather difficult to establish new departments in medical schools. At present, for example, only a few medical schools have independent departments of genetics, even though the science of heredity has clearly emerged as one of the most important fields in all of science, and is of fundamental significance for medicine. Thus, it is not surprising that only a handful of schools have established departments of behavioral science. We believe that such departments will become both more numerous and more diverse in the next decade. We can envision three model departments: behavioral biology, human development, and social medicine. Speaking briefly, the intellectual center of gravity of the first type would be biological, the second psychological, the third social. We believe all three should be vigorously explored; all three will be most rewarding if thoroughly interdisciplinary; and all three should place considerable emphasis on research methods. The presence of such departments in schools of medicine would provide a basic resource not only for psychiatry but for other areas of medicine as well.

It is likely that regional resources will increasingly be needed to deal effectively with psychiatric and other medical-social problems. For example, the new community mental health center program provides many opportunities for tackling important psychiatric problems, but it is not reasonable to expect that strong research competence can be built up in most of these centers in the foreseeable future. There is simply not enough research talent to go around. Therefore, it would be helpful if some of the universities and other research facilities could serve as regional resources for community mental health centers, providing continuing assistance in planning and conducting research in whatever way might be needed. Many intriguing clinical innovations and possibilities for investigation are noted by workers in these centers. What they need is expert consultation and assistance, particularly in problems of method. Similarly, the pooling of information from a variety of centers may be necessary to get adequate data on certain problems. Such pooling might well be effectively coordinated by a regional research center. Also, some types of rather expensive research might best be concentrated in a few strategic locations, with equitable provision for access by investigators at a distance. Models in physical and life sciences already exist. These regional resources could benefit, for example, from the experience of the Brookhaven and Argonne Laboratories, and from the seven Regional Primate Research Centers sponsored by the National Institutes of Health. The Primate Centers have shown a commendable, growing interest in behavioral problems and so have considerable experience of high relevance to the task of psychiatric research.

In the social sciences, economics has pioneered in the formulation and collection of statistical information adequate to its tasks. Now that mental health efforts are being undertaken on a systematic, large-scale basis, a stronger statistical base will be necessary. In the next decade or two, the following sorts of mental health statistics will be sought: cross-sectional and trend data on characteristics of patients utilizing specific psychiatric services, responses to various types of therapeutic intervention, psychiatric case registers, early case-finding techniques, and instruments for achieving reliable classification of patients by diagnostic and socioeconomic criteria. Furthermore, efforts will be made to determine the true prevalence and incidence of specific mental disorders, to link psychiatric records with records from the census, to assess severity and duration of illness in various population groups, to determine the pathways to psychiatric help used by various groups, and to study the relation of life crises to a wide range of medical conditions. These data will make it possible to specify the rates at which different population groups manifest various mental disorders, suffer disability or mortality, and achieve various degrees of recovery. This information is beginning to be collected now in model field stations of the National Institute of Mental Health; it will help assess therapeutic and preventive effectiveness. To plan and organize such data collection systems, it will be necessary to recruit and train a large number of psychiatrists, statisticians, epidemiologists, and social scientists who can work cooperatively.

In the collection of such data, careful attention must be devoted to maintaining the privacy of individuals. Such information should be protected rigorously by laws dealing with privileged communications. Furthermore, data originally collected by one agency for research purposes must never be available to another agency for other purposes. A recent large-scale study of juvenile delinquency demonstrated how personal information can be obtained with adequate safeguards. For example, all information obtained was codified by number and names were not used. It was possible to obtain data without in any way jeopardizing individuals. (For further consideration of this problem, see *The Behavioral and Social Sciences: Outlook and Needs.*)

Fortunately, funds for support of young investigators have been reasonably available as psychiatric research has gradually gained momentum in the 1950s and 1960s. The influx of fresh talent has been essential in creating a new climate for the field. Both private foundations and the federal government have recognized this crucial need and responded wisely. For example, the Small Grant Program of the National Institute of Mental Health has been particularly helpful in getting promising investigators launched. This program deserves strong future support. Here as elsewhere, however, serious warning signals have lately arisen. Federal funds have generally become less available. While this situation has many risks for scientific progress, they are perhaps greatest for young investigators. This risk is heightened by the fact that private foundations have diminished their support for research over the past decade in the expectation that government funds would meet the needs. Today, new funds from private foundations are urgently needed to support workers new to the field.

In this connection, institutional grants can be most helpful. Even a small amount of fluid funds available to a school or department can make a critical difference in the encouragement and aid of talented young workers. Often such people can be recognized locally before they become visible nationally. The opportunity to taste early accomplishment in a locally supported, small-scale project can make a crucial difference in the commitment of a young person to a scientific career. Since the attraction and development of excellent scientific talent has such vital importance for this field, we turn now to a general consideration of this topic.

ATTRACTION AND DEVELOPMENT
OF PSYCHIATRIC SCIENTISTS

Only in the past few years has psychiatry been viewed by scientifically minded students as a field with dynamic research opportunities. If the field is to take advantage of these opportunities, it will be necessary to attract young people of extraordinary quality who perceive the serious nature of the problems and the possibility that scientific tools may solve them. We need to draw talented medical students into psychiatry, but we must also arouse the interest of college and even high school students. One of the best ways to elicit interest in bright, inquiring young people is to give them an opportunity for direct participation before their career intentions have crystallized. Summer work-study projects have proved stimulating for promising young people in high school, college, and medical school. Such opportunities in mental health research should be expanded. College experiences along this line often set the stage for later interest and competence in psychiatric research.

The day may not be too far off when good high schools will provide useful introductions to behavioral science. Such courses would be valuable not only in attracting scientifically minded students to these fields, but more generally in providing the basis for a rational attitude toward the understanding of human behavior and its problems. We hope that government agencies, professional organizations, and universities will strengthen their present efforts to prepare accurate, attractive curricular materials for such courses. It is essential that leading workers in psychiatry and other behavioral sciences take part in the preparation of such materials.

At more advanced levels, there is evidence of strong interest in behavioral science among college students, many of whom are interested in possible careers in mental health professions. One difficulty for such students—and indeed a general problem in today's world of long, complex, technical preparation for careers—is considerable uncertainty about the nature of these professions. What, for instance, does a psychiatrist actually do in his day-to-day work? How many different kinds of psychiatric careers are there? What are the probable gratifications and problems in each career line?

Work experiences in psychiatric settings can be helpful in answering these questions. Such work experiences should be made readily and visibly available to college students, with consistent supervision and instruction provided—in laboratories, clinics, hospitals, and community health centers. Some colleges have well-organized volunteer programs, as well as part-time employment programs, that provide a channel to such experiences. They not only facilitate exploration of possible career interests, but also tap students' deep motivation to help fellow human beings in distress. We hope that joint ventures of students, faculty, and administration can provide many more opportunities of this sort in the near future. We are confident that the psychiatric profession will respond warmly to such ventures.

In schools of medicine and their associated hospitals, exposure in depth to basic concepts and methods of behavioral science is becoming increasingly important for medical students, psychiatric residents (engaged in clinical specialty training), and residents in some other areas of clinical medicine, especially pediatrics. Recent studies in the United States and England have documented the need for strengthening this aspect of medical education.

Until recently, medical schools were generally not strong in the teaching of clinical psychiatry and psychiatric research. Even today, a discrepancy is notable between the importance of psychiatric problems and the adequacy of preparation to meet them in general medical education. This lag is particularly evident in regard to psychiatric research. An NIMH program providing modest stipends for medical students to work on summer projects has been helpful, but this program is badly in need of strengthening. This is one area where modest additional support is likely to have strong impact. The medical school years are particularly important because the interest and skill developed at that time can so readily provide the "launching pad" for long-term contributions.

Since research in psychiatry has developed more recently than that in most other medical fields, it is especially important for medical students to come into close contact with effective psychiatric investigators. Indeed, today many medical students have very little awareness of the ways in which behavioral science research is relevant to medicine. There are many steps that can be taken to improve this situation by scientifically oriented departments of psychiatry. These include presentation by faculty and visitors of ongoing research; opportunities for interested students to meet with such speakers to pursue questions in depth and to gain personal acquaintance with distinguished scientists; meetings of incoming students with advanced students who are active in research to gain the special perspective of peer learning. Above all, interested students must have the opportunity to participate with faculty members in research, with the student receiving adequate supervision and serving in a role in which he is not merely "an extra pair of hands." In psychiatry as in other fields, this will require greater flexibility of curriculum than has usually existed in medicine. Fortunately, the current national trend in medical education is toward greater individuality, thus facilitating the pursuit of special interests. This enhances opportunities for research to be incorporated as a vital part of the educational experience—not restricted to those who wish to puruse research careers, but readily available as a general enrichment for medical education.

In the decade from 1945 to 1955, the scientific aspects of psychiatry were not vigorously pursued within the field, even though considerable financial support was available. The number of scientists recruited and developed within the discipline was small. Some leaders urged young psychiatrists to defer all research activities until they had accumulated many years of clinical experience. It was widely believed that research productivity in this field could occur only late in life. Many believed that no special training was needed for psychiatric research—only clinical experience and mature reflection. Some even maintained that research was trivial altogether, that it was unnecessary or impossible, or both. These attitudes, while still present, are now much less commonly held. The obstacles in the path of the young psychiatrist who has a serious interest in research are less formidable than in that earlier era.

In recent years, we have seen the emergence of scientifically oriented psychiatric departments and institutes that make a special effort to attract young people who show exceptional promise for scholarly leadership in psychiatry. Recognizing the varying backgrounds, talents, and interests of individuals, these departments are striving for a diversity of career outcomes—teaching, research, administration, public service, and private practice. In psychiatric specialty training, these departments are trying to cultivate a sense of personal involvement with the field as a scholarly discipline and to instill a sense of obligation toward its advancement.

A primary objective of these educational programs is to encourage the lifelong study of human behavior in the light of evidence from relevant behavioral and biological sciences. In their clinical specialty training, they tend to facilitate the development by each resident of an area of special competence. This requires sufficient curricular flexibility and scientific guidance to permit the resident to explore in depth some important problem. By the third year of the residency (or sooner), each resident becomes a resource person in his problem area, not only for his fellow residents but for the faculty as well. Such areas of special competence often figure importantly in his later career.

To pursue this type of psychiatric education, it is necessary to emphasize multiple individual pathways through the residency, with careful monitoring to assure that all residents attain basic competence in the core skills and substantive material of clinical psychiatry and its scientific basis. The residency program cannot present a fixed and immutable body of knowledge. Rather, its emphasis should be on learning to keep abreast of clinical and scientific developments in the field as they occur over the years. All psychiatrists will require critical ability to assess new developments. Those who do research will require additional skills.

At the present time, only a few psychiatric residency programs emphasize research training, but many additional centers, particularly in major universities, are making new efforts in this direction. In the leading programs, characteristically, research has a high priority in the values of the faculty; effective models of research competence are readily available to young psychiatrists; and a high proportion of applicants are "research prone," in the sense of having prior research interests, lively curiosity, and exceptional intellectual capacities. Such residencies tend to emphasize teaching in terms of evidence in clinical as well as basic matters. They encourage questioning, emphasize the need for first-hand observations (such as patient interviews), and teach scientific method in relation to psychiatric problems. Usually, they build on a broader base of biobehavioral science than has been traditional in the field. We believe that such residencies hold great promise for advancing psychiatric knowledge and competence.

One of the difficult issues facing such programs is how they can provide real substance in diverse areas, giving the resident at least a useful introduction to biological, psychological and social approaches. For those residents who are serious about research, a good deal more is required than of most other residents. An introduction to the related sciences is not sufficient; depth is required. This means that specialists in the related fields should have an active participation in the training program. Indeed, as we have noted, the modern scientifically oriented departments of psychiatry are increasingly providing a home base for a variety of behavioral and biological scientists. In this sense, psychiatric research has become remarkably broad in its interests. These nonpsychiatric scientists in departments of psychiatry not only conduct research and enrich psychiatric training programs; they also bring along a new generation of students in biobehavioral sciences who are more aware of psychiatric problems and at home in psychiatric settings than their predecessors. Increasingly, too, the scientists—both psychiatrists and nonpsychiatrists—in such departments are centrally involved in decision-making, such as the selection of residents and the formulation of curriculum.

Unfortunately, modern, scientifically oriented departments of psychiatry, of which we have here sketched some prominent features, are still in short supply. Yet long-term progress in the field rests heavily on such departments. Their promise has implications for several groups. For universities, they can serve as a model in department-building—not for all universities, but for those that have a strong commitment to utilizing science in the service of man. For government agencies and private foundations interested in the scientific base of psychiatry and solution of the most difficult psychiatric problems, such departments deserve a very high priority. For scientifically oriented students, especially in medicine, such departments offer exceptional, diverse opportunities.

Psychiatry has had little experience in promoting the career development of those who are likely to spend a substantial portion of their time in research over many years. In the psychiatric education of such individuals, it is useful to distinguish between the residency period and the postresidency fellowship period, both of which can contribute greatly to career development in terms of integrated clinical and research competence. Research preparation can and should be a part of the residency for those who show high-level research promise. However, such people will in most cases need additional fellowship experience in order to develop the complex skills required in modern research.

The two-year period that follows the residency is a crucial one. At this time, promising investigators may easily be lost because there are important factors operating against pursuit of an academic career at a time when the individual typically does not have an established reputation and is particularly uncertain of his ability to make research contributions. It is important that postresidency fellowships be available to provide favorable conditions for seeing the promising man through this critical period. Such conditions include intellectual stimulation, research guidance, academic role models, interpersonal supports, and adequate stipends. Stipends for postresidency fellows have consistently been much too modest.

Sustained personal contact with an effective scientist is crucial in this stage of development. Such contact may lead to a kind of preceptorship in which there is a close working relation between faculty member and fellow. The pattern of joint effort may vary from occasional consultation to intensive supervision, from virtually complete freedom to detailed guidance, and all manner of collaborative relations may evolve. There is no universal prescription for fruitful faculty-fellow relations; here again, individualization is a wise course.

In the postresidency fellowship (and in the junior faculty years), it is important for the young investigator to be able to devote a large proportion of his time to research. There is a tendency for fellows and young faculty members to be drawn into other activities (clinical, administrative, and teaching) on such a large scale that they cannot devote themselves to the exacting demands of research competence. However, in most cases it will not be advisable to exclude all other activities, since some diversification is likely to be stimulating and helpful in long-range career development.

The development of careers that emphasize research in psychiatry and closely related fields has been outstandingly facilitated by far-sighted programs of the National Institute of Mental Health. Beginning with the pioneering Career Investigator Program, proceeding through the various Research Career Development programs, and recently culminating in the innovative Research Scientist Program, these efforts have been remarkably successful. They surely deserve strong continuing support. In our view, they rank with the outstanding career development programs in all of science.

Unfortunately, the Psychiatry Research Training Program, administered by the Psychiatry Training Branch of NIMH, has not enjoyed comparable success. Most university departments and teaching hospitals have not applied. The program has not been well known. The stipends have been quite unrealistically low. Though intentions have been constructive, the program has in effect had low priority of staff and review committees over many years. Yet the concept is basically sound, and speaks directly to the critical shortage of research manpower within our short scientific tradition. The time is ripe for invigoration and upgrading of this program.

In a newly emerging field of scientific endeavor, fraught with difficulty, one type of helpful stimulus is the provision of awards and prizes at all levels of experience. We are encouraged to note that some departments, schools, and professional organizations have taken such steps, particularly for younger investigators. The American Psychiatric Association has set an admirable example with its Hofheimer Research Award. Over the years, this award has been given to relatively young investigators from various disciplines who have done research of high quality pertinent to psychiatric problems. Basic science and clinical investigations have been included. We hope that this example will be followed in a variety of settings, both inside psychiatry and beyond it.

In the development of professional careers that emphasize research competence, the social environment is of crucial long-term significance. Where will the investigator find understanding, appreciation, recognition, and support during his long period of preparation which must include much uncertainty and some disappointment? What conditions favor the breaking of new scientific ground? How can we foster the talent that can solve central problems of human suffering? This is an immense challenge, not just for one profession, or for the scientific community, but for the whole society.

CONCLUDING COMMENT

We must emphasize that the encouraging trends we have sketched in this book represent an early stage in the development of research on psychiatric problems. We have been more concerned with the solution of psychiatric problems than with any proprietary position regarding psychiatry as a profession. Among other effects, we hope that this book will help to attract more talented young people to enter the various behavioral sciences and mental health professions. We can think of no problems more poignant in their human impact, more urgently in need of solution, or more pertinent to the social concerns of our time.

What has been accomplished so far in moving toward solution of these problems of fear, hate, violence, and desperation is only a start. Most of it has been achieved by a relatively small number of scientists and clinicians in a few fields working for a rather short time. Although there were, as we have noted, pioneering contributions in earlier times, the scientific study of human behavior on substantial scale is largely a product of the mid-twentieth century. If these pages indicate promise, there is surely a long road to fulfillment.

Psychiatry today is moving on many fronts to meet its broad social responsibilities and to take advantage of its distinctive scientific opportunities. Central to this effort are three commitments: a searching, constructively critical self-appraisal within the discipline; an enhanced readiness to work closely with scientists of other disciplines—biological, medical, psychological, and social; and a determination to attract and develop top-notch research talent toward work on psychiatric problems. Now as never before in history, the strengths of science are being mobilized to solve problems of emotional distress, personal disintegration, and human relationships.

SELECTED
REFERENCES

Chapter 1

For a general textbook of psychiatry, see Frederick C. Redlich and Daniel X. Freedman, *The Theory and Practice of Psychiatry* (New York: Basic Books, 1966). See also Jack R. Ewalt and Dana Z. Farnsworth, *Textbook of Psychiatry* (New York: Blakiston Division, McGraw-Hill, 1963). See also Lawrence C. Kolb, *Noyes' Modern Clinical Psychiatry*, 7th ed. (Philadelphia: W. B. Saunders, 1968).

For a very comprehensive, detailed textbook prepared by many authors, see Alfred M. Freedman and Harold I. Kaplan, eds., *Comprehensive Textbook of Psychiatry* (Baltimore: Williams and Wilkins, 1967).

For a statement of the scope of mental health problems and a social perspective on mental disorders, see John A. Clausen, "Mental Disorders," in Robert K. Merton and Robert A. Nisbet, eds., *Contemporary Social Problems*, 2d ed. (New York: Harcourt, Brace & World, 1966), pp. 26–83.

For an extensive statement of recent trends in psychoanalysis, prepared by many authors, see Judd Marmor, ed., *Modern Psychoanalysis: New Directions and Perspectives* (New York: Basic Books, 1968).

For a concise overview of psychoanalysis, see Douglas D. Bond, "Some Perspectives on Psychoanalysis," *American Journal of Psychiatry* 122 (1965): 481–84.

For a concise review of recent progress in mental health services, see Alvin Becker, N. Micheal Murphy, and Milton Greenblatt, "Recent Advances in Community Psychiatry," *New England Journal of Medicine* 272 (1965): 621–26, 674–79.

For an extensive account of mental health services with emphasis on social science contributions, see Morris S. Schwartz et al., *Social Approaches to Mental Patient Care* (New York: Columbia University Press, 1964).

For a conceptual framework for social and community psychiatry, see Melvin Sabshin, "Theoretical Models in Community and Social Psychiatry," in *Community Psychiatry*, ed. Leigh M. Roberts, Seymour L. Halleck, and Martin B. Loeb (Madison: University of Wisconsin Press, 1966). Reprinted in paperback (New York: Anchor Books, Doubleday, 1969).

For a recent account of community mental health services, prepared by a variety of authors, see Leopold Bellak and Harvey Barten, eds., *Progress in Community Mental Health*, Vol. I (New York: Grune & Stratton, 1969).

For a review of one major mental health problem, prepared for the general reader, see *Alcohol and Alcoholism* (Washington, D.C.: U.S. Government Printing Office, Public Health Service Publication No. 1640, n.d.).

For a symposium on relatively rigorous assessment research on the effectiveness of services, see Ernest M. Gruenberg, ed., "Evaluating the Effectiveness of Mental Health Services," *Milbank Memorial Fund Quarterly*, Vol. 44 (1966). 402 pages.

Chapter 2

For an introduction to research in schizophrenia, prepared for the general reader, see *Research in Schizophrenia* (Washington, D.C.: U.S. Government Printing Office, Mental Health Monograph No. 4, n.d.).

For a comprehensive review of research and clinical problems in schizophrenia, see C. Peter Rosenbaum, *Understanding Madness: Phenomenology, Sociology, Biology, and Therapy of the Schizophrenias* (New York: Science House, 1970).

For a summary of family studies and genetic studies by the investigators, see David Rosenthal and Seymour S. Kety, eds., *The Transmission of Schizophrenia* (New York: Pergamon, 1968).

For a psychosocial research approach in schizophrenia, see Lyman C. Wynne and Margaret Thaler Singer, "Thought Disorder and Family Relations of Schizophrenics," *Archives of General Psychiatry* 9 (1963): 191–98.

For an interdisciplinary symposium of recent research on schizophrenia, see John Romano, ed., *The Origins of Schizophrenia* (Amsterdam and New York: Excerpta Media Foundation, 1967).

For a concise summary of biochemical research on schizophrenia, see Seymour S. Kety, "Current Biochemical Approaches to Schizophrenia," *New England Journal of Medicine* 276 (1967): 325–31.

For a comprehensive review of depression, see Aaron T. Beck, *Depression: Clinical, Experimental, and Theoretical Aspects* (New York: Hoeber Medical Division, Harper and Row, 1967).

For a research monograph on behavioral aspects of depression, see Roy R. Grinker, Sr. et al., *The Phenomena of Depressions* (New York: Hoeber, 1961).

For a study of the scope of depressive problems, see Charlotte Silverman, "The Epidemiology of Depression: A Review," *American Journal of Psychiatry* 124 (1968): 883–91.

For an introduction to certain aspects of brain chemistry pertinent to depression and schizophrenia, see Solomon H. Snyder, "New Developments in Brain Chemistry: Catecholamine Metabolism and the Action of Psychotropic Drugs," *American Journal of Orthopsychiatry* 37 (1967): 864–79.

For more detailed reviews of biochemical and pharmacological evidence in the context of depression, see Joseph J. Schildkraut and Seymour S. Kety, "Biogenic Amines and Emotion," *Science* 156 (1967): 21–30. See also Joseph J. Schildkraut, "The Catecholamine Hypothesis of Affective Disorders: A Review of Supporting Evidence," *American Journal of Psychiatry* 122 (1965): 509–22. See also William E. Bunney, Jr., and John M. Davis, "Norepinephrine in Depressive Reactions: A Review," *Archives of General Psychiatry* 13 (1965): 483–94.

For an effort to utilize basic research findings in the study of depressed patients, see James W. Mass, Jan Fawrett, and H. Dekirmenjian, "3-Methoxy-4-Hydroxy-Phenylglycol (MHPG) Excretion in Depressive States: A Pilot Study," *Archives of General Psychiatry* 19 (1968): 129–34.

For basic research conducted in psychiatry with a view toward long-range clinical significance, see Alan M. Steinman, Stanley E. Smerin, and Jack D. Barchas, "Epinephrine Metabolism in Mammalian Brain after Intravenous and Intraventricular Administration," *Science* 165 (1969): 616–17.

For reviews of endocrinological research in depression, see James L. Gibbons, "The Adrenal Cortex and Psychological Distress," in Richard P. Michael, ed., *Endocrinology and Human Behaviour* (London: Oxford University Press, 1968). See also Jan A. Fawrett and William E. Bunney, Jr., "Pituitary Adrenal Function and Depression, An Outline for Research," *Archives of General Psychiatry* 16 (1967): 517–35.

For a classic study of grief, see Erich Lindemann, "Symptomatology and Management of Acute Grief," *American Journal of Psychiatry* 101 (1944): 141–48.

For an analysis of psychological factors pertinent to depression, see Frederick T. Melges and John Bowlby, "Types of Hopelessness in Psychopathological Process," *Archives of General Psychiatry* 20 (1969): 690–99.

For a preventive approach to disorders of childhood, see Leon Eisenberg, "Preventive Psychiatry," *Annual Review of Medicine* 13 (1962): 343–60.

For a review and analysis of research on childhood problems by various investigators, see Stella Chess and Alexander Thomas, *Annual Progress in Child Psychiatry and Child Development, 1968* (New York: Brunner/Mazel, 1968).

For a comprehensive review of research and clinical observations on attachment behavior, as well as a theoretical analysis of instinctive behavior, see John Bowlby, *Attachment and Loss*, Vol. I, *Attachment* (New York: Basic Books, 1969).

For a concise account of several research frontiers in child development research, see Alberta Engvall Siegel, "Current Issues in Research on Early Development," *Human Development* 12 (1969): 86–92.

For a sociological and psychiatric study based on long-term followup, see Lee N. Robins, *Deviant Children Grown Up* (Baltimore: Williams & Wilkins, 1966).

For a landmark study in social psychiatry, see August B. Hollingshead and Frederick C. Redlich, *Social Class and Mental Illness* (New York: Wiley, 1958).

For a comprehensive review of the scope of depressive problems, see Charlotte Silberman, *The Epidemiology of Depression* (Baltimore: Johns Hopkins Press, 1968).

Chapter 3

For a comprehensive, critical review of current psychopharmacology, see Donald F. Klein and John M. Davis, *Diagnosis and Drug Treatment of Psychiatric Disorders* (Baltimore: Williams & Wilkins, 1969).

For a concise review of controlled studies of the most widely employed drugs in treatment of depression and schizophrenia, see John M. Davis, "Efficacy of Tranquilizing and Antidepressant Drugs," *Archives of General Psychiatry* 13 (1965): 552–72.

For a discussion of methods in psychopharmacology research see Leo E. Hollister and John E. Overall, "Methodology for the Clinical Investigation of Psychotherapeutic Drugs," *Journal of New Drugs* 5 (1965): 286–93.

For a comparison of various approaches to treatment of depressed patients, see Milton Greenblatt, G. H. Grosser, and H. Wechsler, "A Comparative Study of Selected Antidepressant Medications and EST," *American Journal of Psychiatry* 119 (1962): 144–53.

For a review and analysis of methodological progress and clinical research results, see Martin Katz and Jonathan Cole, "Research on Drugs and Community Care," *Archives of General Psychiatry* 7 (1962): 345–59.

For a review of the effectiveness of major tranquilizers in acute schizophrenia, see The National Institute of Mental Health Psychopharmacology Service Center Collaborative Study Group, "Phenothiazine Treatment in Acute Schizophrenia," *Achives of General Psychiatry* 10 (1964): 246–61.

For a study of one of the newest promising developments in psychopharmacology, see William E. Bunney, Jr. et al., "A Behavioral-Biochemical Study of Lithium Treatment," *American Journal of Psychiatry* 125 (1968): 499–512.

For comprehensive reviews of recent research on psychotherapy and suggestions for future inquiry, see Hans H. Strupp and Allen E. Bergin, "Some Empirical and Conceptual Bases for Coordinated Research in Psychotherapy: A Critical Review of Issues, Trends, and Evidence," *International Journal of Psychiatry* 7 (1969): 18–90. See also Allen E. Bergin, "Some Implications of Psychotherapy Research for Therapeutic Practice," *International Journal of Psychiatry* 3 (1967), 136–50.

For a large-scale effort at pooling information on psychoanalytic practice, see David A. Hamburg et al., "Report of the Ad Hoc Committee on Central Fact Gathering Data of the American Psychoanalytic Association," *Journal of the American Psychoanalytic Association* 15 (1967): 841–61.

For a review of current research on psychotherapy, mainly derived from the disciplines of psychology and psychiatry, see Allen T. Dittman, "Psychotherapeutic Processes," *Annual Review of Psychology* 17 (1966):

51–78. See also Donald H. Ford and Hugh B. Urban, "Psychotherapy," *Annual Review of Psychology* 18 (1967): 333–72. See also Rosalind Dymond Cartwright, "Psychotherapeutic Processes," *Annual Review of Psychology* 19 (1968): 387–416.

For interdisciplinary perspectives on psychotherapy by a variety of investigators, see Hans H. Strupp and Lester Luborsky, eds., *Research in Psychotherapy*, Vol. II (Washington, D.C.: American Psychological Association, 1962). See also Eli A. Rubinstein and Morris Parloff, eds., *Research in Psychotherapy* (Washington, D.C.: American Psychological Association, 1959).

For a concise review of evidence on the role of expectation in the outcome of psychotherapy, see Jerome D. Frank, "The Influence of Patients' and Therapists' Expectations on the Outcome of Psychotherapy," *British Journal of Medical Psychology* 41 (1968): 349–56.

For research on rehabilitation of patients with relatively severe disorders, including the chronically hospitalized, see Denise Bystryn Kandel and Richard Hays Williams, *Psychiatric Rehabilitation, Some Problems of Research* (New York: Atherton Press, Prentice-Hall, 1964).

For a comprehensive review and analysis of research on group dynamics and group therapy, see Irvin D. Yalom, *The Theory and Practice of Group Psychotherapy* (New York: Basic Books, 1970).

Chapter 4

For research pertinent to primate experimental models of human disorders, based on laboratory and field observation, see the following publications: B. M. Foss, ed., *Determinants of Infant Behavior*, Vol. IV (London: Methuen, 1969). (In this book, see especially the papers by Harry F. Harlow and Margaret K. Harlow; Robert A. Hinde; I. Charles Kaufman and Leonard A. Rosenblum; and David A. Hamburg.) See also Jules H. Masserman, ed., "Animal and Human," in *Science and Psychoanalysis*, Vol. XII (New York: Grune & Stratton, 1968). (In this book, see especially the papers by Gordon Jensen and Ruth A. Bobbitt; Jules Masserman, Stanley Wechlsin, and Marvin Woolf; and William A. Mason.) See also Phyllis C. Jay, ed., *Primates, Studies in Adaptation and Variability* (New York: Holt, Rinehart & Winston, 1968). See also Irven DeVore, ed., *Primate Behavior, Field Studies of Monkeys and Apes* (New York: Holt, Rinehart & Winston, 1965). See also Allan M. Schrier, Harry F. Harlow, and Fred Stollnitz, eds., *Behavior of Nonhuman Primates, Modern Research Trends*, Vol. II (New York: Academic Press, 1965).

For a recent study of isolation-rearing in chimpanzees, see Corbett H. Turner, Richard K. Davenport, and Charles M. Rogers, "The Effect of Early Deprivation on the Social Behavior of Adolescent Chimpanzees," *American Journal of Psychiatry* 125 (1969): 1531–36.

For a review of hormonal effects in early life upon later behavior in animals, see Seymour Levine and Richard Mullins, "Hormonal Influences on Brain Organization in Infant Rats," *Science* 152 (1966): 1585–92.

For studies of the influence of male sex hormone on aggressive behavior in monkeys and men, see Richard P. Michael, ed., *Endocrinology and Human Behavior* (London: Oxford University Press, 1968). (In this book, see especially the papers by Robert W. Goy; and by John Money and Anke A. Ehrhardt.)

For a review of studies of children's learning of aggressive behavior by observing models in action, see Albert Bandura, "Vicarious Processes: A Case of No-Trial Learning," in *Advances in Experimental Social Psychology*, Vol. II, ed. Leonard Berkowitz (New York: Academic Press, 1965).

For a concise review of major trends of evidence and theory on human aggressive behavior, see Marshall J. Gilula and David N. Daniels, "Violence and Man's Struggle to Adapt," *Science* 164 (1969): 396–405.

For a clinical study of some aspects of violent behavior, see John M. Macdonald, *Homicidal Threats* (Springfield: Charles C Thomas, 1968).

For an extensive review and analysis of human violence, prepared by a group of psychiatrists and psychologists for the general reader, see David N. Daniels, Marshall F. Gilula, and Frank M. Ochberg, *Violence and the Struggle for Existence* (Boston: Little, Brown, 1970).

For a review of the effects of psychological stress on hormones of the adrenal gland, see David A. Hamburg, "Plasma and Urinary Corticosteroid Levels in Naturally Occurring Psychologic Stresses," in *Ultrastructure and Metabolism of the Nervous System*, ed. Saul R. Korey, Alfred Pope, and Eli Robins (Baltimore: Williams & Wilkins, 1962), pp. 406–13.

For review of evidence and charting of new research directions linking genetics with endocrinology and behavior, see David A. Hamburg, "Genetics of Adrenocortical Hormone Metabolism in Relation to Psychological Stress," in *Behavior-Genetic Analysis*, ed. Jerry Hirsch (New York: McGraw-Hill, 1967), pp. 154–75. See also David A. Hamburg and Donald T. Lunde, "Relation of Behavioral, Genetic, and Neuroendocrine Factors to Thyroid Function," in *Genetic Diversity and Human Behavior*, ed. J. N. Spuhler (Chicago: Aldine, 1967), pp. 135–70.

For a symposium on biological approaches to the study of emotional responses, including brain mechanisms, endocrine system, and autonomic nervous system, see David C. Glass, ed., *Neurophysiology and Emotion* (New York: Rockefeller University Press and Russell Sage Foundation, 1967).

For a concise statement on brain and emotion, see Karl H. Pribram, "The New Neurology and the Biology of Emotion," *American Psychologist* 10 (1967): 830–38.

For a comprehensive review and analysis of stress effects upon various endocrine glands in monkeys, see John W. Mason et al., "Organization of Psychoendocrine Mechanisms," *Psychosomatic Medicine* 30 (1968): 565–808.

For a study of surgical patients, centering on fear-arousing aspects of the situation and ways of coping with it, see Irving L. Janis, *Psychological Stress, Psychoanalytic and Behavioral Studies of Surgical Patients* (New York: John Wiley, 1958).

For a classic study of psychological reactions in wartime life-threatening situations, see Roy R. Grinker, Sr., and John P. Spiegel, *Men Under Stress* (Philadelphia: Blakiston, 1945).

For a comprehensive review and analysis of behavioral science literature on stress and coping, see Richard S. Lazarus, *Psychological Stress and the Coping Process* (New York: McGraw-Hill, 1966).

For a major review and theoretical reformulation pertinent to the development of effective coping behavior, see Robert W. White, "Motivation Reconsidered: The Concept of Competence," *Psychological Review* 66 (1959): 297–333.

For clinical observations and reflections on the mastering of stressful experience in personal development, see Erik H. Erikson, *Identity, Youth and Crisis* (New York: W. W. Norton, 1968). See also Robert W. White, *Lives in Progress*, 2nd ed. (New York: Holt, Rinehart & Winston, 1966, paperback). See also Lois B. Murphy et al., *The Widening World of Childhood* (New York: Basic Books, 1962).

For studies of ways in which some normal adolescents cope with their problems, see Roy R. Grinker, Sr., Roy R. Grinker, Jr., and J. Timberlake, "A Study of 'Mentally Healthy' Young Males (Homoclites)," *Archives of General Psychiatry* 6 (1962): 405–53. See also Daniel Offer and Melvin Sabshin, *The Psychological World of the Teen-Ager, A Study of Normal Adolescent Boys* (New York: Basic Books, 1969).

For a concise review of coping behavior in various stressful experiences, see David A. Hamburg and John Adams, "A Perspective on

Coping Behavior: Seeking and Utilizing Information in Major Transitions," *Archives of General Psychiatry* 17 (1967): 277–84.

For clinical studies of persons coping with difficult experiences, see Therese Benedek, "Climacterium: A Developmental Phase," *Psychoanalytic Quarterly*, Vol. 19 (1950). See also Grete Bibring et al., "A Study of the Psychological Processes in Pregnancy and of the Earliest Mother-Child Relationship: I. Some Propositions and Comments," *Psychoanalytic Study of the Child* 16 (1961): 9–24. See also Stanley Cobb and Erich Lindemann, "Coconut Grove Burns: Neuropsychiatric Observations," *Annals of Surgery* 117 (1943): 814–24.

For a broad summary of sleep research, prepared for the general reader, see *Current Research on Sleep and Dreams* (Washington, D.C.: U.S. Government Printing Office, Public Health Service Publication No. 1389, n.d.).

For a concise statement of work on one of the main research frontiers in sleep, see Michel Jouvet, "The States of Sleep," *Scientific American* 216 (1967): 62–72.

For research on sleep in depressed patients, see Frederic Snyder, "Electrographic Studies of Sleep in Depression," in *Computers and Electronic Devices in Psychiatry*, ed. Nathan S. Kline and E. Laska (New York: Grune & Stratton, 1968).

For major reports of current biological and clinical research in sleep, see William Dement, Peter Henry, Harry Cohen, and James Ferguson, "Studies on the Effect of REM Deprivation in Humans and in Animals," in *Sleep and Altered States of Consciousness*, ed. Seymour Kety, E. Evarts and H. Williams (Baltimore: Williams & Wilkins, 1967), pp. 456–68. See also William Dement et al., "Hallucinations and Dreaming," in *Perception and its Disorders*, ed. David Hamburg, Karl Pribram and Albert Stunkard (Baltimore: Williams & Wilkins, 1970).

For a computer analogy to sleep and dreaming processes, see Christopher Evans, "Sleep and Dreaming—A New, 'Functional' Theory," *Trans-Action* (December 1967), pp. 41–45.

For research at the interfaces between biological and social science, see P. Herbert Leiderman and David Shapiro, eds., *Psychobiological Approaches to Social Behavior* (Stanford: Stanford University Press, 1964).

Chapter 5

For a broad, authoritative survey of the behavioral sciences with suggestions for future progress, see *The Behavioral and Social Sci-*

ences: Outlook and Needs. (Englewood Cliffs, N.J.: Prentice-Hall, 1969).

For an introduction to psychiatric research methods, see *Some Observations on Controls in Psychiatric Research* (New York: Group for the Advancement of Psychiatry, 1959), G.A.P. Report No. 42. See also Peter Sainsbury and Norman Kreitman, eds., *Methods of Psychiatric Research: An Introduction for Clinical Psychiatrists* (London: Oxford University Press, 1963).

For a multidisciplinary survey of research on major psychiatric problems, see Derek Richter, J. M. Tanner, Lord Taylor, and O. L. Zangwill, eds., *Aspects of Psychiatric Research* (London: Oxford University Press, 1962). See also Alec Coppen and Alexander Walk, eds., *Recent Developments in Schizophrenia: A Symposium* (Ashford, Kent: Headley, 1967), *British Journal of Psychiatry,* Special Publication No. 1. See also Alec Coppen and Alexander Walk, eds., *Recent Developments in Affective Disorders* (Ashford, Kent: Headley, 1968), *British Journal of Psychiatry,* Special Publication No. 2.

For a concise statement on systematic, large-scale collection of information needed to clarify certain mental health problems, see Morton Kramer, "Mental Health Statistics of the Future," *Eugenics Quarterly* 13 (1966): 186–204.

For survey and analysis of the prospects for psychiatry and behavioral science in medical education, see L. W. Earley et al., eds., *Teaching Psychiatry in Medical School* (Washington, D.C.: American Psychiatric Association, 1969). See also *Royal Commission on Medical Education, 1965–68, Report* (London: Her Majesty's Stationery Office, 1968).

For discussion of newer trends in the training of psychiatrists, see *Training the Psychiatrist to Meet Changing Needs* (Washington, D.C.: American Psychiatric Association, 1963). See also David A. Hamburg, "Recent Trends in Psychiatric Research Training," *Archives of General Psychiatry* 4 (1961): 215–224.

For the student seeking an introduction to psychiatry as a clinical profession, see National Commission on Mental Health Manpower and American Psychiatric Association, *Careers in Psychiatry* (New York: Macmillan, 1968).

For a survey of mental health manpower in relation to contemporary professional trends, see Franklyn N. Arnhoff, Eli A. Rubinstein, and Joseph C. Speisman, eds., *Manpower for Mental Health* (Chicago: Aldine, 1969).